The
FLOURISHING
WOMAN

Dr Cate Howell is a GP, therapist, researcher, educator and author. She has over 40 years of training and experience in the health sphere, and is passionate about the areas of mental health, wellbeing and counselling. Currently Cate is mostly involved in education and writing related to these areas.

Cate holds a Bachelor's in Applied Science (Occupational Therapy), a Bachelor of Medicine, a Bachelor of Surgery, a Masters in Health Service Management and a Doctor of Philosophy (Medicine). She also has a Diploma in Clinical Hypnosis and has trained in a range of therapies.

She has travelled internationally to present research findings and has been published in a number of academic journals. The author of five books, Cate was awarded a year 2000 Churchill Fellowship related to the study of anxiety and depression, and the Order of Australia Medal in 2012 for services to medicine, particularly mental health, and to professional organizations.

The FLOURISHING WOMAN

A mental health and wellbeing guide

DR **CATE HOWELL**

OAM, CSM, CF

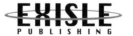

EXISLE PUBLISHING

First published 2023

Exisle Publishing Pty Ltd
PO Box 864, Chatswood, NSW 2057, Australia
226 High Street, Dunedin, 9016, New Zealand
www.exislepublishing.com

A CiP record for this book is available from the National Library of Australia

ISBN 978-1-922539-64-9

Designed by Bee Creative
Typeset in PT Serif, 10.2pt
Printed in China

This book uses paper sourced under ISO 14001 guidelines from well-managed forests and other controlled sources.

10 9 8 7 6 5 4 3 2 1

Disclaimer

This book is a general guide only and should never be a substitute for the skill, knowledge and experience of a qualified medical professional dealing with the facts, circumstances and symptoms of a particular case. The nutritional, medical and health information presented in this book is based on the research, training and professional experience of the author, and is true and complete to the best of their knowledge. However, this book is intended only as an informative guide; it is not intended to replace or countermand the advice given by the reader's personal physician. Because each person and situation is unique, the author and the publisher urge the reader to check with a qualified healthcare professional before using any procedure where there is a question as to its appropriateness. The author, publisher and their distributors are not responsible for any adverse effects or consequences resulting from the use of the information in this book. It is the responsibility of the reader to consult a physician or other qualified healthcare professional regarding their personal care. The intent of the information provided is to be helpful; however, there is no guarantee of results associated with the information provided.

Note from the author

The material in this book has been informed by my decades of experience as a GP and counsellor, and some of the foundational concepts have been covered in my other work, most recently *The Changing Man*. The importance of these strategies in achieving and maintaining good mental health and wellbeing relate to everyone, and as such you may also see them in several of my other books.

To my mother, Marguerite,
and all the amazing women in my life.

Contents

Dealing with issues across the lifespan

Introduction

The Flourishing Woman is all about thriving in life. Flourishing is strongly influenced by our mental health and wellbeing, as well as having a sense of belonging and fulfilment in life. But we are all aware that, at times, it is very hard to have a sense of 'flourishing', especially when life throws challenges in our path.

Our mental health and wellbeing have been especially challenged during the COVID-19 pandemic, and there is a need for information and support right now. This need is evident in therapy practices across the world, in conversations between women, and in the media. *The Flourishing Woman* has been, in part, written in response to this need.

It was also written for another important reason. As women we are probably more used to supporting family members, friends or colleagues, rather than looking after ourselves. Take a moment to reflect on plane travel. At the start, a flight attendant will instruct us to put on our own oxygen mask before we help others. There is a reason for this — if we become low in oxygen, we will not be able to help!

The same can be said in life generally. If we don't care for ourselves, we cannot care for others. This approach is not selfish. We need to prioritize our mental health and wellbeing, including self-care, and take the much-needed time and steps to do this. We will then see the benefits for ourselves and for our loved ones.

My hope is that *The Flourishing Woman* provides some of the information, support and practical 'keys' that might assist you to do just this. No matter where you are starting in terms of your mental health and wellbeing, the aim is to move towards flourishing in life.

The why!

Working for many years as a general practitioner, therapist and educator, I have learnt a great deal by working with many women in my practice and by teaching. Women come to therapy or to educational events seeking information and wanting to achieve change. They may be at a crossroads in some aspect of their lives, or want to experience less anxiety, improved mood, a greater sense of purpose or more satisfying relationships.

Having written a book on men's mental health called *The Changing Man*, I started to wonder whether there might be a need to write a book specifically for women. When I spoke at a Country Women's Meeting in 2021 and asked the group about whether they saw a need for a book focusing on women's mental health and wellbeing, there was a resounding 'yes' from the whole group.

The next realization came when I looked to see what was already out there on the subject. I was surprised to find a few textbooks for professionals but very little for women in general. There was a gaping hole out there, and this needed to be addressed! So here we are, with a book specifically on mental health and wellbeing for women, and also for those who care about them, including family, partners or professionals.

There are many other reasons for *The Flourishing Woman*. Recent research has provided new information that is important to our understanding of mental health and wellbeing. This year I had the opportunity to attend a course at the South Australian Health and Medical Research Institute and learnt about their research on mental wellbeing. They have identified that mental illness and mental wellbeing are *not* two ends of a single spectrum, with health at one end and illness at the other. Mental illness and mental wellbeing are, in fact, two separate but inter-related continua, and the aim is to have a high level of mental wellbeing and a low level of illness.[1] We can do this by focusing on ways to improve or maintain our mental health and wellbeing, and also by recovering from or preventing mental illness. This research has also inspired my focus on wellbeing in this book.

Research has also highlighted the importance of understanding the influence of our neurobiology. We all have billions of brain cells, and as neuroscientist Dr Sarah McKay points out, the connections between these cells are continually 'flourishing', to meet our needs and to enable us to respond to our environment. This means that our brains are plastic and have the potential to change, no matter what our stage in life. We can make use of this potential to recover from issues and to thrive.[2]

Being a woman can be both wonderful and challenging. We have unique capabilities and strengths, and fulfil a range of roles in life, contributing to family, community and workplaces. We also experience a range of challenges, including health-related issues, both mental and physical. For example, we may experience reproductive health issues over our lifespans, and women have higher rates of some health conditions.[3]

There are other challenges. Gender inequality in relation to representation and pay levels persists, and women continue to undertake most household and childcare responsibilities including the related and often hidden mental work.[4] This potentially includes being the main organizer in the home, and remembering a whole array of information related to a partner or family, including special occasions and children's activities.

Women's safety, in and out of the home, continues to be a major and unacceptable issue, with many impacts on women's lives. It is time for society to tackle this. On an individual level, we are seeing women stand up, speak out and be heard and generate the necessary response in the community.

It is also time for us to focus on our own mental health and wellbeing, to place ourselves higher up our priority list, and to have the support and strategies to achieve positive change and personal growth. *It is time to flourish.*

Who, how and what?

When contemplating writing this book, I asked Facebook followers to post about topics they wanted to see included. Again, there was a resounding response. Suggestions included writing about common mental health issues such as anxiety and depression, and many wanted information about hormonal influences and mental health across the lifespan, especially around menopause. There were other suggestions to include dealing with resentment and managing the workload and stress related to 'being all things to all people'. All of these topics, and more, have been included in the various chapters of the book.

The Flourishing Woman is written for adults of all ages and looks at a range of issues affecting women across their lives, in a comprehensive and accessible way. It aims to fill the gap by providing not only information about mental health, but also many practical strategies and ideas about how to achieve a greater sense of wellbeing. For ease of reading, the pronouns she and her will be used in the book.

At the same time my hope is that it provides a compassionate voice and support as we reflect on the different topics. The writing process is quite involved, and despite much experience professionally and personally in life, I found I made discoveries and developed insights as I wrote. We really are travelling on a journey together throughout the book.

The book can be read from start to finish or dipped in and out of as needed. The twelve chapters can work together, but they can also be read as stand-alone chapters. Questions related to vital issues are answered, such as why women so often put themselves last, how to deal with distressing emotions, how to manage change in life, and eating issues, as well as how to silence any internalized critical voice (the 'inner critic') and grow self-compassion.

We will look at challenges faced during the different stages of life that may compromise mental health and wellbeing, and consider strategies to deal with these, and at the same time strengthen our wellbeing. Topics such as reproduction, menopause and mental health, relationship issues, the impact of abuse and trauma on mental health, and a whole range of other issues will be addressed.

Recently I changed my practice logo to a door. Seeing a therapist or undertaking education is all about opening a door to knowledge, understanding, support, change or realizing potential. We are all very familiar with doors, to our homes or workplaces, our favourite coffee shop or a friend's house. Similarly, I think we can all relate to having a door open or close to us in life, as that is life! *The Flourishing Woman* has also adopted this symbol, and hopefully the book will open a door to a conversation about women and mental health and wellbeing. The information provided may well open the door to understanding, validation and a greater sense of empowerment. It may open the door to identifying a range of options for the future. Equally, a door may represent something blocking us, like fear, or be about setting boundaries or closing a chapter in *life*.[5] **Above all, a door may offer hope, a beginning or a gateway to possibilities and change.** Within each chapter, there are brief information boxes with doors, signifying an important piece of information to consider.

There are also keys in the book, which represent practical strategies to open a door or help manage a particular issue. This book is about connecting with ourselves, in terms of awareness and understanding, and using our own valuable resources. It is also about connecting with others, and is a practical guide, focusing on how to enhance mental health and wellbeing, and deal with any mental health issues.

When reading the various chapters, it may be useful to have a notebook or a journal to write down thoughts or feelings along the way. And various questions will be posed and ideas provided to contemplate. Again, thoughts about these could be written in the journal. Let's call it 'the flourishing journal' or 'the journal' for short!

Maintaining health and wellbeing involves addressing our physical, emotional and social wellbeing. We need to feel safe and secure in life and have a sense of belonging and connection. A holistic or 'whole person' approach also takes into account cultural and gender identity, occupations and spiritual life. In therapy, what is called 'an integrative approach' works well. This involves considering all the different aspects of a person and their distress, and combining various therapies to assist. This approach is useful as 'one size does not fit all' and it allows us to tailor therapy to each unique individual.

The Flourishing Woman is written using an integrative approach. It draws on recent studies that have discerned which psychological interventions are most effective in improving women's mental health and wellbeing. For example, there is evidence that mindfulness-based and positive psychological interventions are very effective in improving mental health, and other approaches (such as Cognitive Behavioural Therapy or Acceptance and Commitment Therapy) can also have positive effects.[6] More about these approaches later!

When?

Our mental health and wellbeing are vital to a satisfying and meaningful life. This book is all about working with your thoughts, feelings and actions to increase your sense of health and wellbeing so you can deal with the unexpected occurrences that life throws at us at times. Sometimes we experience distressing but normal reactions to stressful situations, and understanding these reactions can be helpful.

We all develop knowledge and many resources during our lifetimes that can support our mental health and wellbeing. Despite terrible adversity during World War II, Anne Frank held onto hope, and her words have continued to inspire the world. In her diary, Anne wrote, 'everyone has inside of her a piece of good news. The good news is that you don't know how great you can be, how much you can love, what you can accomplish, and what your potential is.'[7] *The Flourishing Woman* is about using all of our resources to reach our potential.

Together, we will tap into our own expertise, stories and resources, and review useful information and practical strategies along with the odd piece of wisdom! Let's be inspired to find the keys and to open the doors together to greater awareness and connection with ourselves and with others, to change and possibilities, and to continuing to develop our skills to improve our mental health and wellbeing. Thank you for being here as we explore and grow together. It's time to flourish!

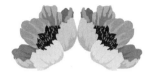

LET'S OPEN THE DOOR TO FLOURISHING

Understanding women's mental health and wellbeing

"

Be there for others, but never leave yourself behind.

— Doldinsky

The aim of this chapter is to open the door to greater understanding about the mind and women's mental health and wellbeing issues in general. We will start with some definitions, current ideas about mental health and wellbeing, and some facts and figures. We will also explore ways to protect our mental health, and answer some of the potential questions about common mental health problems and what causes them.

First let's consider the story of Mary, who was the 'rock' in her family and struggled to care for herself.

Mary's husband and adult children relied heavily on her, and she spent most of her time looking after everyone else. Over time she found herself feeling more and more tired and 'worn down'. She said that she felt irritable and was teary at times. Mary loved to garden and to walk the family's dog, Blackie, on the beach. She also liked to visit her friend, Lena, who lived a few hours away. But these things weren't happening very much at all and Mary's mental health was suffering.

We will come back to Mary's story a bit later.

This chapter covers not only important information to be aware of at the outset but it also addresses the question: Why, as women, do we so often put ourselves last? This question will get you thinking about your priorities and your own life. We also consider a few practical strategies for prioritizing ourselves more. Plus, the chapter contains a whole range of ideas to consider and provides the first of many keys to wellbeing and flourishing.

To start, a few definitions

Let's look at some definitions so that we can understand the language used in our community around mental health and wellbeing. We'll then take a look at the words we'll use throughout the book.

Both physical and mental health are vital to our sense of overall wellbeing. The term **mental health** is often misunderstood. Sometimes it is equated with illness, but it is about feeling healthy and having a sense of **wellbeing**. Mental health reflects our psychological and social wellbeing and has been defined as a state in which you realize your potential, can cope with various stresses in life, can work productively, and contribute to the community.[1]

Recent research has suggested that mental health and wellbeing means we can better manage our mood, stress and anxiety levels. It also includes life satisfaction (or whether we like the life we lead),[2] 'positive' emotions, meaning and purpose in life, resilience, character strengths, and interpersonal relationships.[3] This is why we will take a broad look at mental health and wellbeing and incorporate all of these aspects into our approach.

Resilience refers to our ability to adapt during challenging times.[4] It has been particularly important in recent years with the pandemic and natural disasters. We all need resilience to manage change, setbacks and our emotions. This is why many of the approaches and strategies in the book foster resilience.

And, as indicated by the title of the book, we are very much focusing on **flourishing**. This has been defined as thriving, and has been adapted by the field of positive psychology to living a 'good life' or, in other words, finding fulfillment, meaning and connection.[5]

Flourishing refers to thriving in life, or finding fulfilment, meaning and connection.

The terms **mental illness** or **mental disorder** are commonly used to refer to a diagnosable illness that 'affects a person's thinking, emotions and behaviours, and disrupts the person's ability to work or carry out daily activities and engage in satisfying personal relationships'.[6] On the other hand, **mental health problem** is a broader term related to having symptoms not severe enough to be diagnosed as an illness, possibly following a life crisis, and causing significant distress.[7]

Let's consider physical health for a moment. We can be a physically healthy person generally, but unwell when we catch a virus. Let's apply this to mental health. As mentioned earlier, recent research has provided new insights into mental health. There is evidence that mental illness and mental health are *not* two ends of the same continuum (a line with a range low to high) as once thought. In other words, we can have mental health and wellbeing *and* experience mental illness at the same time.[8] And importantly, these continua are inter-related, which means we can work on our wellbeing even if there is mental illness; and that improving our mental health and wellbeing can assist in recovery from mental illness, help with prevention, and also help us to grow and flourish in life.

Improving our mental health and wellbeing helps us to flourish.

Facts and figures about women's mental health

Part of focusing on wellbeing is understanding some of the potential mental health problems that can influence wellbeing, and learning how to prevent or manage them. The following facts and figures set the scene on potential problems and we will address some of these later in the book.

» Depression is common worldwide, with approximately 280 million people experiencing it.[9] Rates of depression vary between countries, but it is reported that it occurs twice as commonly in women as men.[10]

» In 2019, over 300 million people were living with an anxiety disorder.[11] Women are said to be two to three times as likely as men to be impacted by anxiety disorders, including generalized anxiety disorder and panic disorder.[12]

» Some women experience disorders at times of hormone change, for example, around the birth of a baby, premenstrually or around menopause (addressed in Chapter 8).

» Women who have experienced childhood trauma are several times more likely to develop depression as adults (see Chapter 10).[13]

» Mental health issues are commonly reported by lesbian, gay and queer women.[14]

» The prevalence of severe mental illness is reported to be higher in women, and the co-occurrence of more than one mental health problem (comorbidity) is also observed more frequently among women.[15]

» 80 per cent of people with eating disorders are women, and 26 per cent of young women have self-harmed (twice the rate of young men).[16] (See Chapter 7.)

A recent study showed that the COVID-19 pandemic has increased rates of anxiety and depression in the community generally. This was found to be related to the pandemic's effects on work, finances and our social lives. These were strongly associated with increased mental health symptoms and decreased psychological wellbeing.[17]

A women's health survey in 2022 also indicated a decline in mental health, especially in young women. The survey reported that 17 per cent of women with a pre-existing mental health issue said their mental health had worsened.[18] We will talk more about the effects of the pandemic on mental wellbeing in Chapter 5.

Some mental health problems are reported to occur more often in women. The COVID-19 pandemic has had a significant impact.

Why are the rates higher in women than men?

There are many potential reasons for the reported higher rates, but we must not ignore the evidence that women are often placed in a more vulnerable position in society, whether being seen as inferior, suffering more stress, or being subjected to abuse or violence.[19] These factors will have a significant impact on mental health.

It is also suggested that even though we tend to talk about our issues, we may still internalize some emotions (such as anger). We also tend to go to the doctor fairly regularly in the Western world in relation to reproductive issues or with children, so we may be more likely than men to speak with a doctor about our mental health at the time.

Women are also more likely to be diagnosed with a mental health disorder even in situations where men have the same scores on mental health assessments and are not diagnosed. Plus, we are also more likely to be prescribed medication.[20] This raises questions and concerns about potential biases in terms of diagnosis and treatment based on gender.

What are the causes of mental health problems?

Our mental health and wellbeing is influenced by many and varied things, from genetic tendencies to an illness, to what we eat and what we do in life. Both mental wellbeing and mental illness result from interactions between the mind, body and environment. In practice we talk about a 'multidimensional' or 'bio-psycho-social' basis to maintaining mental health and wellbeing and understanding problems which might arise.[21] Cultural and spiritual or other factors may also be relevant.

Let's consider a few examples of 'bio-psycho-social' influences on mental health and wellbeing. Biology includes our genetics, physical illnesses, nutrition, hormonal influences or drugs/medications. Some illnesses may be inherited genetically from our parents; vitamin deficiencies or thyroid conditions may cause mental health issues, or alcohol or substance use may be related.

Psychological influences include stress (such as stress caused by a heavy workload), personality factors (e.g. tending to have a more obsessional or perfectionistic nature), our sense of safety and security, early styles of 'attachment' to caregivers (see p. 240) or experiences of neglect, abuse or trauma. Social factors include financial stress or poverty, lack of social supports, housing issues, violence and migration.[22] Stigma and discrimination in relation to gender and sexuality may contribute.

It is also important to look at causes of mental health issues through different lenses, which can help us to find focus. For example, a gender lens highlights the importance of psychological distress caused by hardship, abuse or exploitation, which have been shown to impact women's mental health. These may be compounded by inequalities related to culture, age or sexuality.[23]

Risk and protective factors for our mental health

We talk about factors that protect our mental health and those that put us more at risk. This is useful because as individuals and as communities, we want to reduce risk factors and enhance the protective factors. Many strategies to enhance our mental health and wellbeing are based on this.

We need to focus on reducing risk factors for mental health problems, and growing our protective factors for mental health and wellbeing.

In 2019, a large study on risk and protective factors for mental wellbeing was carried out, and the factors were found to include the following:[24]

Risk factors	Protective factors
Social isolation and loneliness	Strong social relationships
Homelessness	Physical activity
Being in a sexual minority	Employment
Migration	Nutrition
Cyberbullying	Alcohol reduction
Insecure employment and unemployment	Access to nature (green space)
Unsupportive work conditions	
Economic inequality	
Caregiving	
Physical health conditions	
Stressful life events (including violence or natural disasters)	

In addition, the study found that for women around the time of giving birth, risk factors to mental wellbeing include childhood and lifetime abuse, chronic medical conditions, stress and unsupportive relationships, disturbed sleep and multiple births. Social support and physical activity are protective.

Note that strong social relationships or social connectedness, or lack of it in terms of isolation or loneliness, are listed under protective and risk factors. Social connections are vital to our wellbeing. American trauma expert Dr Bruce Perry writes that 'We are social species; we are meant to be in community — emotionally, socially and physically interconnected with others'.[25] Writer and journalist Johann Hari has suggested that a significant cause of depression is 'Lost Connections'.[26]

There will of course be variation in how much social connection we each need, depending on our personalities.

Connection is a vital key: Connection to others is vital to our mental health and wellbeing. We need to find a level of connection that works for us as individuals.

It is important to recognize any **warning signs** for mental health problems. These include:

» persistent sadness or feelings of hopelessness

» excessive fear or worry

» changes in eating or sleeping habits, appetite or weight

» low energy and fatigue

» extremely high and low moods

» increased irritability

» social withdrawal

» misuse of alcohol or drugs

» suicidal thoughts.[27]

Please be alert for these and seek assistance if they are evident (this is essential if there are suicidal thoughts; see Chapter 7).

The value of different 'lenses'

As alluded to earlier, it is useful to view mental health, mental illness and related psychological approaches through different 'lenses'. A lens can help us focus or see different perspectives. We have already mentioned a gender lens; let's now consider a few other lenses.

Mental illness is often viewed through a 'disease' lens. This can be helpful in identifying the problem and providing assistance, but there can be risks of labelling too early or in error. A more recent lens involves a 'process-based' framework, in which the problem a person is experiencing is seen as potentially being made up of a 'network' of issues. For example, if the person is depressed, there may be a range of issues related to loss or loneliness.[28] A more process-based approach also incorporates the idea that there are common processes maintaining different problems, and we need to deal with them. An example would be catastrophic thinking, which may be shared between different types of anxiety or depression[29] (addressed in Chapters 4 and 6).

A helpful lens is the humanistic lens, which emphasizes individuality, and the person's own perspective. An early psychological approach called Gestalt sees the person as having much expertise, as does narrative therapy. The existential lens focuses on the value of meaning and purpose in life. The cognitive-behavioural lens considers the impact of our thoughts and behaviours on how we feel.

Trauma is very common in our community. Psychiatrist Dr Bruce Perry uses a lens of 'What happened to you? or 'What didn't happen for you?' rather than 'What is wrong with you?'[30] This is an example of adopting a trauma-informed lens, as trauma so often contributes to the development of mental health problems. Perry suggests that sometimes trauma and its effects are missed and, as a result, an incorrect diagnosis can be made.[31]

In this book we'll tap into a number of lenses, but the main lens will be the holistic view already mentioned. This recognizes that there are many facets to ourselves and our lives. It sees the importance of addressing illness when present, and also focuses on developing our mental health and wellbeing so that we can flourish in life. Additionally, an individualized and compassionate approach to mental health and wellbeing is seen as vital.

It is important that we are heard and respected, and seen as having many resources within us.

Why do we put ourselves last?

To flourish, we need to ensure that we prioritize our mental health and wellbeing, but it is a common experience for women to struggle with this. An Australian National Health Survey of Women found that 'women are trying to do too much or they think they're expected to do so much'.[32]

Women learn to nurture their children and family, and often their needs come first. This is often necessary, but putting others first and ignoring our own needs may cause harm. Family and the society in which women live both influence women's lives. Society is viewed broadly as being made up of family, friends, school, government, media, culture, religion and more! We have all been influenced in positive and negative ways, and women are often trained to look after everyone else first. This can result in a sense of wanting to please others most of the time.

People-pleasing can also arise from the multiple demands on us, or experiences of trauma and the stress response that results. This is why we often struggle to say 'no' to demands. However, frustration or resentment can result when we are exhausting ourselves trying to meet all these demands. Difficulty saying 'no' may be involved. What can then result is taking on too many tasks and not including enough rest or time-out in the week.

Women are often raised to put themselves last and look after everyone else first. This can result in wanting to please others, which can come at a cost.

In addition, as humans, we naturally compare ourselves to others. **Comparison** is one of our innate survival mechanisms to keep us safe. In the modern world, comparison and a sense of lack (we are somehow lacking in beauty, body or something else in life) is fostered by media and advertising, principally to sell products to us. Social media excels in this as it commonly focuses on 'the perfect woman'. This mystical creature leads to unrealistic ideals and contributes to a lot of harm in our society for women. A good way to remember to drop comparison is to recognize that to compare means to despair!'

At the centre of women not prioritizing themselves can be a sense of being less important than, or being 'less than', others. As we grow up, we naturally create stories in our minds about ourselves. Some are on track but others are not. Unfortunately, a 'not enough' story about ourselves can develop. We will talk more about this story in Chapter 3, but right now it's important to recognize that we are valued and 'enough', and our wellbeing matters.

You are enough: Work on changing the 'not enough' story into 'I value myself, and I am enough'.

Prioritizing mental health and wellbeing

Remember the example of plane travel and oxygen masks on p. 1? This highlighted the need to prioritize our mental health and wellbeing, including self-care. This approach will benefit ourselves and those for whom we care.

In this section, we will consider one of the major barriers to self-care for women, and that is time! And we will look into related issues such as self-belief, setting boundaries and assertiveness (which can assist us to say 'no') in Chapters 3 and 7. It can be challenging to give ourselves time, and some women are in situations where it is incredibly hard to do this.

For some women, making the decision to focus on what they value can help. We only have so much time and energy in life and need to focus these in areas that are most important to us. Let's hear more about Mary for a few moments:

> Mary recognized that something needed to change. She spoke with her good friend, Lena, who suggested that she see a counsellor regularly.
>
> Mary started making a few changes. She let her family know that she needed some time to herself and would be spending regular

quiet time in the garden or walking the dog. Mary also made the commitment in her mind to visit Lena more often. With these changes, she found her mental wellbeing started to improve.

Sometimes, finding time can come through cancelling some activities in the diary or reducing tasks at work. Learning to have more boundaries and to be more assertive may be related to the time issue. For others it is recognizing that we can't solve everyone else's problems and that they actually need to learn to do this for themselves. Teaching others that we practise self-care and won't always be available to care for their needs may play a role.

To flourish, prioritize mental health and wellbeing: This may mean allocating more time for yourself by checking in on what is most important to you in life and letting others solve their own issues wherever possible!

Another interesting idea is 'work–life integration'. This is about finding ways to blend different areas of life to improve wellbeing. For example, if you travel by train to work, walking to and from the station each day can provide some regular exercise. Having boundaries about not checking any emails after the end of the formal workday enables more relaxation or time to spend time with your partner or family. However, finding time might not be so straightforward, particularly if you have significant social or financial constraints. We achieve change by taking small or 'baby' steps, starting with just one. It may be that the first step is accessing some support from a therapist or community organization for help in making some changes.

Take steps to prioritize self-care: Small changes in what you do, think or say can bring big rewards. And having support in making these changes can help.

 ## Let's summarize

Mental health and wellbeing refer to a state in which everyone realizes their own potential, can manage various stresses, contributes and has a sense of belonging. It is all about flourishing!

We can work directly on improving our wellbeing, and sometimes we need to address any mental health problems impacting our wellbeing. *The Flourishing Woman* addresses both.

We may experience a range of mental health issues and are more vulnerable at times of hormonal change. There can be many related factors, such as biological, psychological or social factors. Women are often placed in more vulnerable positions in life and violence remains a significant issue. Homelessness is a growing issue in our communities. In addition, COVID-19 has had a large impact on women's mental health and wellbeing (see Chapter 5).

A holistic, individualized approach to working with mental health and wellbeing is vital. Recognizing the strengths and resources already within us can assist, along with focusing on a healthy lifestyle, self-care and connection with others.

Discussion about an important question was included in this chapter, namely why women so often put themselves last. There are complex reasons for this, but we can begin to prioritize ourselves more by taking small steps towards self-care.

Let's summarize the keys from this chapter. Remember, too, that by prioritizing our wellbeing, and maybe seeking some support to do so, we can work towards flourishing.

» Connection is a vital key.

» We are enough.

» To flourish, prioritize mental health and wellbeing.

» Take steps to prioritize self-care.

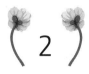

The foundations of mental wellbeing and flourishing

It isn't where you came from; it's where you're going that counts.

— Ella Fitzgerald

This chapter focuses on general ways to support and improve our mental health and wellbeing. It has been a challenge to write about ways to both grow wellbeing *and* manage mental health issues. Both are vital, and this chapter provides a foundation to addressing both.

You are the expert on yourself and once you are aware of the various steps to support and grow your mental health and wellbeing, you can make choices that fit best for you. My clients often run with these, as shown in Rani's story:

Rani was a relatively new mother and was feeling very anxious. When we talked about all the changes that had happened in Rani's life during the last eighteen months (including a move interstate) and identified that the anxiety was the result of these changes, she understood that her reaction was pretty 'normal' given the circumstances.

Rani was also expecting a lot from herself, so we looked at some ways to manage those expectations along with the anxious feelings, including meditation, and Rani ran with all of this. She also organized childcare once a week so that she could return to a yoga class and catch up with a friend.

This chapter continues to increase our awareness, not only about mental health and dealing with life issues, but also about how our mind actually functions. Our brain cells have the potential to grow and form new connections and nerve pathways to meet our needs (known as **neuroplasticity**). An example is learning a new language — we focus and practise, and over time our mind creates new pathways so that we can understand and speak the language.

The brain is amazingly 'plastic!' Our brain cells have the potential to form new connections throughout life, so that we can learn and flourish.

The Flourishing Woman is based on our capacity to learn, change and adapt to life's challenges. This chapter, which outlines ten potential foundational steps to improve mental health and wellbeing, is based on neuroplasticity and learning new skills.

First, a few words about prevention

A good level of mental health and wellbeing can help us feel good and enjoy life, and can also assist in preventing mental health problems. Prevention strategies may focus on reducing risk factors such as poor nutrition, substance use, stress, trauma or social isolation, and improving some of the protective factors such as healthy lifestyle, connecting with others and doing meaningful activities in life.

Positive Psychology, which was originally developed by Martin Seligman, has a lot to offer in relation to prevention. This field of psychology moved away from focusing on illness and instead focused on character strengths and behaviours, with the aim of helping people thrive. Seligman has a wellbeing theory that highlights the roles of experiencing 'positive' emotions (such as joy or love), engagement in life and activities, relationships, meaning in life, and accomplishment. This approach focuses on developing skills for healthy relationships, utilizing mindfulness, self-care and a range of coping skills. **Mindfulness** is a process of awareness, and involves paying attention on purpose, to experience the present moment as opposed to being caught up in thoughts or feelings.[1]

It is in a mindful state that the nerve cells in the brain are activated and growth is stimulated.[2] That is, being mindful enables neuroplasticity and is now considered particularly beneficial to many aspects of our mental health and wellbeing. This is why we will incorporate mindfulness in various places throughout this book.

Mindfulness involves paying attention with our senses, on purpose and without judgment. It provides a powerful way to grow new nerve cell connections in the brain, and to strengthen our resilience and wellbeing.

Positive Psychology also considers the role of values and being authentic in life, and fostering a sense of purpose, meaning and hope.[3] Authenticity is about being genuine in relation to who you are and how you live. Living more authentically means having self-awareness and skills to live authentically (e.g. to not be overly influenced by others). Note that a specific therapy, positive therapy, has arisen from this approach.

The aim of Positive Psychology is not for us to have 'happy' thoughts and feelings all the time, as this is not possible — in fact we naturally have a 'negative bias', or tendency towards negative thinking, to help us survive. However, we do know that our wellbeing can benefit from increasing our positive emotional experiences, such as interest, gratitude, inspiration, love or amusement.[4]

The work of researcher Carol Dweck in relation to education has also influenced our thinking on mental health and wellbeing and prevention. She coined the terms 'fixed or growth mindsets' to describe the beliefs that students had about their intelligence and ability to learn. A growth mindset involves beliefs, goal setting and effort to learn and achieve. When you have a growth mindset, you believe you are capable of change, of adapting, and of learning new things. On the other hand, if you have a fixed mindset you believe the opposite

— that you cannot learn anything new, and you cannot change your thinking or your attitudes. Improving mental health and wellbeing and prevention involves adopting a growth mindset.[5]

Strategies from Positive Psychology and positive therapy will be woven throughout the book. Getting to know and use them can help us to flourish.

Ten steps towards mental health and wellbeing

These ten foundational steps are drawn from current thinking and evidence related to achieving optimal brain function and from psychological approaches that strengthen our mental health and wellbeing, and help to address mental health issues.

1. Raise self-awareness and identify what to focus on.

2. Be mindful of your emotions.

3. Choose some intentions or goals.

4. Attend to your physical health, lifestyle and self-care.

5. Connect with others.

6. Tap into talking therapies (to manage thoughts, feelings and behaviours).

7. Know and use your strengths.

8. Explore self-compassion, meaning and purpose.

9. Enjoy meaningful activities and practise gratitude.

10. Consider complementary therapies or medication (if needed to address a mental health issue).

These steps are not in a particular order, and you won't need to necessarily do them all. For some, seeking help might come first, while for others, improving physical health will be the priority. Let's consider one step at a time; you might like to write down any useful ideas in your journal as you go.

1. Raise self-awareness and identify what to focus on

Much of the work we do on our mental health and wellbeing relates to being more self-aware. This includes how physically and mentally healthy we feel, our personality styles, our internal strengths and resources, and how we deal with any challenges or changes in life.

It may be that we are not actually aware of what we think and feel. You might also want to reflect on how connected you feel with yourself and others, and what issues are impacting you at this time. Some concerns might be troubling you more than others or negatively impacting your mental health and wellbeing. These issues may be obvious, but sometimes there are a number of things involved, or they may be hidden (such as the effects of abusive behaviours within relationships). Equally, there may be a network of inter-related experiences, feelings or challenges you are trying to identify and sort out.

Perhaps start by looking at the range of factors that can influence mental health and wellbeing. Physical factors include being tired, not having enough nutritious food, not drinking enough water or being unable to find time to exercise or relax. Equally, using substances or having chronic illness can affect our health.

Emotional factors may be affecting wellbeing, such as feeling stressed, anxious or low in mood. Loss, grief, trauma or anger may be impacting. There may be social issues related to housing, employment, relationship problems or lack of social support or connection. Perhaps there are spiritual concerns, such as questions about what life is about; cultural factors; or sexuality or gender-related issues.

We can open the door to change by reflecting on issues that might be impacting our mental health and wellbeing.

Reflecting on your **values** in life, or what is important to you, can assist in identifying areas to focus on. We can have values in different areas of life such as family and friends, intimate or partner relationships, work and finances, education or personal growth, health and fitness, leisure, the community or environment, and spirituality. Becoming aware of and focusing on what is important to you in these areas can reduce stress and help you find a greater sense of meaning and purpose.

It can be helpful to first identify what is important to you in each of these areas, and then to ask yourself if there is a gap between what you feel is important and what is actually happening. For example, if being physically fit is important to you, and there is no time to exercise, then there is a gap to address. A review of your values in relation to each of the areas of your life and any current gaps could be recorded in your journal.

Sometimes looking at values can lead to surprising outcomes:

Betty came to therapy as she had been feeling depressed. The values exercise led to discussion about her main aim during retirement, which had been to travel. However, at retirement her husband took up an interest that required him to attend to it every day. There were no trips away and she had a large sense of loss. Once this issue came to light, it was possible to look at options for dealing with it, and a session with Betty and her husband led to a good outcome. They would travel some of the time, and their son would look after his father's interest when they were away.

Reflect on your values: We have a more fulfilling life when our actions are aligned with our values. Consider reviewing your values in your journal.

Often, writing enables you to express what is troubling you and leads to new insights. Consider using the journal to write freely about what is happening, or not happening, and any related feelings. Or write a list of the main issues that have come to light and add to it as other issues become apparent. You might also try talking with a trusted family member or friend, or a doctor or therapist to help identify any troubling issues. The ones needing attention more urgently can then be prioritized.

2. Be mindful of your emotions

Emotions or feelings are fundamental in life and reflect our inner state. We can experience a whole range of them each day, and they can vary in intensity and pleasantness. Our individual experience of them can also vary. Emotions can be described in a word, such as ecstatic, sad, despairing, jealous or ashamed, as different from thoughts, which relate to our head-talk and are usually a string of words.

Emotions don't come from just one part of the brain. They come from throughout our brain and body (including the gut). The nervous system is constantly collecting information about our internal and external worlds and making sense of it. A 'core affect' (or emotional state) results, referring to how 'good or bad' we feel in a particular situation.[6]

Emotions are often categorized as 'positive' or 'negative', for example happiness or sadness. This categorization has limitations, but in terms of evolution the more negatively perceived emotions have helped us survive. Author Leonard Mlodinow says that it is useful to start with the idea that the more negative emotions, while unpleasant or distressing, are there to help us recognize conditions that are suboptimal or unsafe, and alert us to make the necessary changes. Without them, we would have little desire to change anything.[7]

Understanding emotions is about being more connected to yourself, and getting to know what is happening in your mind and body.

In terms of our wellbeing, there is a tendency to think that the more 'positive' emotions we have, the better. They are vital as they help us feel good and function well, and they can trigger creativity. However, the whole range of emotions helps us to assess our experiences, and many of life's meaningful experiences include some emotional challenge. These experiences, although not always pleasant, can help us grow as individuals. This is why more recent theories about wellbeing recognize the importance of meaning and personal growth. And one reason why the term 'negative' emotions doesn't always fit. As a result, we are going to refer to them as 'distressing' or 'uncomfortable' emotions.

Much has been written about core or basic emotions, with various models aiming to group all of the many emotions under five to eight headings. Psychologist Paul Eckman proposed a series of universal emotions in humans, based on associated facial expressions. He grouped them into the basic emotions of surprise, sadness, happiness, disgust, anger and fear.[8] It has also been proposed that the basic emotions relate to primitive states of stress (fear, anger), punishment (sadness) or reward (joy).[9]

Recent research by social worker and author Brené Brown found that hundreds of emotions and related experiences were reported. Brown concluded that in order to recognize and make sense of our feelings we need to:

» understand how they show up in our bodies and why

» get curious about how our families and communities shape our beliefs about the connections between our feelings, thoughts and behaviour

» examine our go-to behaviours

» recognize the context of what we are feeling or thinking by asking ourselves, 'What brought this on?'

Brown groups emotions under a range of headings. There isn't space to mention them all, but they include 'places we go' when things are uncertain (e.g. 'overwhelm, anxiety, vulnerability') or when we're hurting ('sadness, grief, despair'); when we fall short ('shame, self-compassion, perfectionism'); when we search for connection ('belonging, insecurity, loneliness'); when the heart is open ('love, heartbreak, trust'); when life is good ('joy, calm, gratitude'); and places we go with others ('compassion, empathy, boundaries').[10]

Let's focus on empathy and vulnerability for a few moments. Empathy is about being aware of, and sensitive to, the experience (the thoughts, feelings) of another person. It is different from sympathy as it involves imagining ourselves in the other person's position, and understanding to a degree what they are going through.[11] Empathy is ultimately about connecting with other people, and is good for our wellbeing. (You can find Brené Brown talking about empathy on YouTube.)

Empathy is about being able to tap into our own experiences in order to connect with the experience of someone else, or to see it from their perspective. It leads to connection.

Empathy may involve vicariously feeling the emotions of the other person. We are able to do this because we have nerve cells in the brain called 'mirror neurons', which create physical sensations and emotions that mirror what the other person is experiencing. Some people struggle with empathy, such as when there are unhelpful beliefs (e.g. blaming victims). Narcissistic personality traits can also lead to a lack of empathy (more on this in Chapter 9).

Brené Brown has done a lot of work on vulnerability. She defines it as 'the emotion that we experience during times of uncertainty, risk, and emotional exposure'.[12] For example, we might experience vulnerability after miscarriage, relationship breakdown, or when a child leaves home. Brown emphasizes that vulnerability is not a weakness. In fact, it takes great courage to go through these times, to feel the feelings and to possibly share them with others.

There is much more to explore about emotions as we go through *The Flourishing Woman*, but a key message is that understanding emotions is about recognizing what is happening within the mind and body. A lot of our distress comes from attempting to suppress or avoid uncomfortable emotions. However, developing awareness, rather than trying to avoid emotions, is the basis upon which we can work with them. This involves mindfulness, as we are not judging the emotions as 'good or bad', simply observing them.

To understand more about emotions: Be mindful and connect with how emotions show up in your body. Where do you feel them? What do they feel like? Recognize how they relate to your thoughts and behaviour.

It is also important to recognize that difficulties can occur when the more distressing emotions continue to dominate, such as in anxiety, depression or potentially with grief, loneliness or anger issues (see Chapters 6 and 7). However, there are many approaches and strategies that can assist, as we will find out as we explore several mental health issues and life challenges in later chapters.

3. Choose some intentions or goals

Once you have identified any aspects of your mental health and wellbeing that you want to work on, or any troubling issues, the next step is to choose some related intentions or goals. We intuitively know how to decide on a goal, but taking the first step can often be the hardest part. As Chinese Philosopher Lao Tzu said: 'The journey of a thousand miles begins with one step.'

The 'why' or the reasons for working on the goal often relate back to your value or what is important to you in different areas of your life. Keeping the reasons and the benefits of the work in the forefront of your mind helps with motivation. For example, reasons for changing a behaviour like smoking might relate to health or money; or seeking help with relationship issues might be motivated by concern for children.

Here is an example to go by when setting some goals. Let's say the issue is feeling flat in mood, and low in energy, and exercise has helped in the past to improve this. Working through the goal might look like this:

» *My goal* is to do more exercise and spend time in nature by walking along the river.

» *My why?* I know that I always feel better in myself when I get some exercise and get out into nature.

» *Steps to achieve my goal* include:
   › working out whether to go alone or with someone
   › planning when to walk, for how long and how often
   › preparing a bag to take with me with a water bottle, sunglasses, my phone and some money in it

> › setting a reminder on my phone and note that I have walked in my diary.

> » *Details and date to achieve this goal by?* Start walking by Saturday this week. I will aim to walk twice a week, then review at one month.

Start with the most achievable goal and work on one goal at a time. Author and researcher B.J. Fogg talks about the idea that we are more likely to achieve change when we take very small steps. He suggests working out what you will do and when you will do it, preferably tying the change into a current habit (e.g. after breakfast). He also suggests celebrating when each step is achieved, and to do this straight away to reinforce the change and create a new 'tiny habit'.[13] Examples of celebrations might be having a great cup of tea or coffee, calling a friend, or doing a celebratory dance! It can also help to write down your goals as well as the steps involved, and then tick off each step as it is achieved. Celebrating works, because a small amount of dopamine (a brain chemical associated with reward) is released in the brain, which helps us feel good and cements the change.

How to work with goals: Keep the 'why' in mind and keep things very simple. Take very small steps and celebrate when each step is achieved!

It can be helpful to reflect on creating some 'happy habits' or 'relaxing habits' to tap into regularly. Happy habits might include connecting with someone, or having a smile or laugh. Relaxing habits might include breathing, meditating or exercising. You can use your journal to write about some of these habits, or to tease out some goals!

4. Attend to your physical health, lifestyle and self-care

Our physical health is central to flourishing. And when our mental health and wellbeing is challenged, it is important to make sure there are no underlying physical problems that may be contributing, for example low iron levels that can lead to tiredness. This is why seeing a doctor regularly for a check-up is recommended; and remember that a check-up can include checks on emotional wellbeing too.

Aim to find a relatable doctor to talk to about any health issues, share any family history of illnesses and discuss lifestyle and self-care. They can work through any current issues such as tiredness, worries or low mood, and check up on sleep, hormonal or related issues. A doctor may utilize assessment tools such as the 'Patient Health Questionnaire-9', the Kessler-10 or the Depression, Anxiety and Stress Scale to further assess mental health and wellbeing. A doctor can also check your blood pressure, do a general physical examination, and organize further investigations if needed. Depending on your age or history, screening tests may be suggested (e.g. blood sugar level tests, cervical or sexually transmitted infection screens, breast checks, electrocardiograph, bone or bowel health tests).

Sometimes health problems such as anaemia, low vitamin D or thyroid issues can trigger emotional issues, and improvements can be felt when these are treated. Chronic illnesses, such as diabetes, or conditions such as Parkinson's disease or sleep apnoea may greatly impact our mental health too.

Have a regular check-up with a doctor: Why not go to the doctor soon and take a list of any concerns and questions so they can be addressed?

It may be useful to complete the Kessler-10 Scale at this stage. Developed in the United States and used worldwide, the scale measures current psychological distress but does not diagnose particular problems. However, a high score on this scale can indicate that there could be issues such as anxiety or depression that need to be checked out further with a health professional. (See 'Resources', p. 333.)

It is important not to underestimate the benefits of lifestyle and self-care to our mental health and wellbeing. Lifestyle measures are not just about feeling good. There is evidence that healthy nutrition and sleep, and regular physical movement benefit our bodies and minds. They can actually foster new brain cell development and optimal brain functioning.[14]

Take some time to consider the following measures to improve mental health and wellbeing through lifestyle changes:

>> Think about ways to connect with other people (family and friends, work colleagues or consider joining a group).

>> Value yourself and value self-care. Drop the idea that self-care is 'selfish'.

>> Eat a variety of healthy foods. Shop around the edges of

the supermarket where all the fresh food is or try a farmer's market for a change.

» Drink at least 2 litres (4 1/4 pints) of water a day. Consider having fewer caffeinated or energy drinks, as they can creep up in number.

» Follow your country's guidelines for alcohol intake.

» If you're a smoker, look at ways to quit. There are often triggers to smoking such as after a meal, which need to be tackled. Hypnosis can be helpful.

» Work on reducing the use of other substances, and get some help if need be.

» Get some regular exercise. Start with small steps and build it up gradually.

» Having a satisfying sexual relationship can influence emotional wellbeing. Recognize that your sex life will vary at different times.

» If sleep is an issue, work on ways to improve it (see p. 147). If need be, have sleep apnoea checked out.

Over halfway there!

» Disconnect from phones, tablets or laptops regularly. Our brain needs time away from being stimulated by technology, and it needs silence too.

» Find time to relax. Pause and do nothing, breathe, listen

to relaxing music or try a relaxation app. Perhaps learn to meditate or try yoga.

» Practise mindfulness in everyday activities (be present in the shower, for example, and notice the sensations), or utilize mindfulness meditation.

» Do more enjoyable, creative or meaningful activities.

» Enjoy some pampering activities, such as having a pot of tea, a hot bath or shower, a pedicure or a massage.

» Get out into nature regularly (go on a forest walk) and feel at peace or in awe!

» Laugh often, as humour de-stresses you. Smiling has a positive effect too!

» Be grateful for the good things that happen in life, as gratitude helps lift mood (see p. 54).

Adopting some of these measures can make a huge difference to our mental wellbeing. Maybe write down a few that seem helpful to you in your journal. Keep them in mind and consider setting a couple of goals related to them.

Do a lifestyle review: Review different aspects of your lifestyle, such as nutrition, exercise, sleep and stress management, and think about a few related goals.

5. Connect with others

As humans, we all need connection with other people. Some people need a great deal of connection while others prefer more limited connection, depending on our personality style. Social connection has been shown to aid our physical and psychological health and our sense of wellbeing. Brené Brown is reported as saying; 'We are ... wired to love, to be loved, and to belong. When those needs are not met, we don't function as we were meant to.'[15] Spending time with or speaking with a trusted person, like a partner, family member or a good friend, is really valuable to our mental health and wellbeing. It helps us feel connected and contributes to a sense of belonging. We can connect with friends or via educational pursuits, community groups, creative or sporting activities or through social media or online forums.

Connection is particularly important when we feel distressed. Simply speaking out loud helps us to express and work through our emotions. And it feels really good to be listened to, understood and validated. Being heard and understood are basic human needs, so think about sharing issues or emotions when the problem feels troubling. You might also reach out to a coach, work colleague, doctor or therapist.

Our lives transform via connection, whether through making friends, meeting partners or connecting with a community group. Here is the story of Vicky, who felt extremely lonely and depressed.

> Vicky had moved to a regional town after a divorce and knew no one in the area. She had one daughter living two hours away. The local mental health nurse talked to Vicky about ways to make connections in the area, but it was actually on the advice of a woman working in the supermarket, who showed kindness and chatted regularly with

Vicky, that she joined a community group and found her 'tribe'. This had very beneficial effects on her life and she didn't need to see the nurse very often any more.

6. Tap into talking therapies (to manage thoughts, feelings and behaviours)

Therapy is based on talking to someone who is trained and skilled, who can help us to understand what is going on in our life. Talking therapies help us utilize our own resources, address any issues and make changes to our thoughts, feelings and actions.

Our understanding of the mind and its neurobiology has influenced modern-day therapies. The brain carries out many functions, from helping our heart to beat, to making sense of what we see and hear. It allows us to relate to others and to come up with creative ideas.

The areas of the brain of interest to us are:

» The brainstem at the top of the spinal cord, which controls basic functions of the body and helps us survive. Stress activates this part of the brain, which then increases our heart and breathing rates. It helps keep us safe.

» The limbic brain (the amygdala and hippocampus), which is responsible for emotions and memory. Trauma is mostly processed in this area, and it has a focus on helping us feel satisfied or content.

» The cortex, which houses language, imagination and awareness, and is responsible for decision-making and judgment. This part helps us connect with others.[16]

However, as author Leonard Mlodinow explains, the different areas of the brain have evolved over time and in fact are all interconnected, and not separate entities. Emotions and different functions occur in different parts of the brain, and these areas communicate and work together.[17] Neurosurgeon Dr Rahul Jandial describes the brain as an ecosystem, like an ocean, with activity and interconnection everywhere.[18]

We have an automatic nervous system that controls much of our survival response. It has 'sympathetic' and 'parasympathetic' arms. The sympathetic arm is responsible for our fight or flight response when we feel threatened. The parasympathetic arm has dorsal vagal nerves, which trigger the freeze response when we are in danger (i.e. we are immobilized or may collapse), and the ventral vagal nerves, which help us feel safe and connected to others (more on this in Chapter 10).

With the discovery of neuroplasticity we have learned that our brains have the capacity to change. We believe this is one of the reasons that talking therapies can help as we are learn new ways of thinking, feeling and behaving. Talking therapies range from counselling to specific psychological approaches.

We will draw on a number of specific therapies throughout the book, including:

» Cognitive Behaviour Therapy (p. 69)

» Acceptance and Commitment Therapy (p. 71)

» Interpersonal Therapy (p. 125)

» Narrative Therapy (p. 71)

» Hypnotherapy (p. 112)

» Dialectical Behaviour Therapy (p. 188)

» Positive Therapy (p. 30).

When seeking help from a therapist, make sure they have sound training, are professional in their approach, and you feel comfortable talking with them. A doctor or relevant professional organizations can help you locate an appropriate therapist.

7. Know and use your strengths

Strengths are positive attributes that reflect our values. They are often called 'values in action'. When we recognize and work with our strengths, we tend to be happier. It can actually be very hard to recognize our strengths when this has not been part of our upbringing. We may have taken on messages growing up to not get too big for our boots, or perhaps we only received negative feedback.

Society also tends to hold ideas about what female strengths 'should' be (e.g. being kind and caring rather than assertive or showing leadership), and these ideas influence us to take on these traits. Some of these ideas are not always helpful — for example, self-sacrifice can come with cost.

However, strengths can be remarkably broad and include assets such as creativity and humour. It is interesting to look at how strengths are classified. They are grouped under six main 'virtues':

1. Wisdom: creativity, curiosity, judgment, love of learning, perspective
2. Courage: bravery, persistence, honesty, zest
3. Humanity: love, kindness, social intelligence
4. Justice: teamwork, fairness, leadership
5. Temperance: forgiveness, modesty, prudence, self-control

6.   Transcendence: appreciation of beauty, gratitude, hope, humour, spirituality.[19]

Take a few moments to reflect on your own potential strengths in your journal, or explore them further through the questionnaire listed in the 'Resources' section on p. 333.

Work with your strengths: Identifying and using your strengths can help you feel more content.

8. Explore self-compassion, meaning and purpose

William Holman Hunt is quoted as saying, 'The door of the human heart can only be opened from the inside'. Self-compassion means that we are kind and understanding towards ourselves when we are having a difficult time, instead of criticizing and judging ourselves harshly.[20] Researcher and author Kristin Neff developed a self-compassion scale, and showed that those who score higher on this scale have greater wellbeing.[21]

Nurturing ourselves via self-compassion gives pleasure and enables us to lift our own spirits. It is associated with happiness, optimism, wisdom, curiosity and emotional intelligence. It can also help us deal with pain, and help relationships.[22] One of the reasons self-compassion can do all of this is that it activates the soothing and calming parts of the nervous system (the ventral vagal system).[23]

> Practising more self-compassion is 'gold' in terms of our mental wellbeing.

Neff has identified self-compassion as having three main elements, namely mindfulness, common humanity and kindness. These must all be present and they interact. We have spoken about mindfulness, and in this context Neff says that we must to turn towards our uncomfortable emotions and acknowledge them. We need to be mindful of them so that we can respond with kindness.[24]

Common humanity refers to recognizing our own humanity. Being connected is part of compassion, both to others and ourselves. We turn inward and acknowledge our imperfections as part of being human, knowing that all humans are worthy of compassion. We then respond with self-kindness. For example, we may have made a mistake and feel guilty, but we can still respond to ourselves with kindness.

We will continue to explore strategies to grow self-compassion in Chapter 3. Let's now consider meaning, which is linked to self-compassion. Studies have shown that people who are more self-compassionate report experiencing a greater sense of 'meaning in life'.[25] So what do we know about meaning and purpose, and why are they important?

Psychiatrist Viktor Frankl (1905–97), one of the founders of Existential Therapy, wrote that the essence of being human could be found in the search for meaning. He described three sources of meaning: a life purpose; a love; and a sense of meaning through suffering. He also suggested that we must be self-aware and focus on something bigger than ourselves.[26] A recent study on meaning by researcher Brodie Dakin explored the theory that meaning involves having a positive, helpful relationship to others. Dakin defined meaning as a combination of our sense of purpose, significance and coherence, with significance relating to viewing our own lives as significant in making positive difference in the lives of others.[27]

Purpose refers to the reason we do what we do, and is also about following our values and doing what we love. Purpose and meaning are inter-related and both can improve our wellbeing and life satisfaction. We may want to help the environment or love caring for animals. Purpose may also be living simply, doing simple acts of kindness when we can, or being creative in some way. It is at these times, too, that we feel in the 'flow' or completely absorbed.

Creating a sense of meaning and purpose improves our wellbeing and sense of fulfilment. It often involves looking outwards, such as helping others.

A useful model to share is the Japanese concept of *ikigai*, which is essentially 'a reason to get up in the morning' or a reason to enjoy life. The model incorporates our 'passion, mission, profession and vocation' or in other words what we love, what we are good at, what the world needs and what we can be paid for. Where all of these overlap is our *ikigai*.[28]

Reflect on ikigai: Consider how 'what you love, what you are good at, what the world needs and what you can be paid for' might come together in your life to create a sense of purpose.

A word of warning here, as not everyone can readily locate their 'why', and that is okay! Sometimes identifying your purpose is a task that takes a lifetime, so instead it might be better to simply focus on getting to know yourself better, being authentic in who you are and how you live, consistent with what you value.

Here are a few ways to connect with your sense of meaning and purpose:

» Be self-aware and reflect — what gives you energy in life?

» Be guided by or what is important to you — possibly family, simplicity in life, looking after the planet, being creative, justice or service.

» Manage time to create space for the things you feel are important in life.

» Practise self-care.

» Connect with others and have helpful relationships.

» Be aware of thoughts that block your purpose, such as 'I couldn't do that'.

» Quit self-criticism, practise self-compassion, and build self-belief.

» Recognize and trust in your strengths and abilities.

» Recognize your right to embody your purpose.

» Be in the moment, and enjoy it!

Mindfulness helps us in many ways, including enjoying the moment. But future thinking is also important in terms of planning and making decisions, which helps us find meaning. There is evidence that future-thinking aids wellbeing. We might imagine how we can help someone in the future, plan simple acts of kindness, or contemplate positive things happening in future life.[29]

9. Enjoy meaningful activities and practise gratitude

Work and leisure involve many activities. These not only provide us with routine and enjoyment but they can also foster a sense of meaning and purpose, and can give us a great sense of satisfaction and achievement. Life can become busy and we may drop activities that give us meaning. Equally, loss of motivation can occur in relation to mental health problems, so it may be harder to engage in usual activities.

We all enjoy different sorts of activities. Some of us enjoy movement such as sport or walking the dog, while others enjoy playing or listening to music or watching movies. Some activities are very social, while some have physical health benefits or incorporate relaxation. Creative pursuits, such as music or art, allow self-expression.

To illustrate the benefits of meaningful activity, here is the story of Mariza:

> Following a stroke, there were many activities Mariza struggled to carry out independently and she was feeling depressed. She was encouraged to engage with an activity that had meaning for her. She chose making something for her son that would be valuable to him. Slowly, but surely, this was achieved, when the task was completed she smiled broadly and took it away to give to her son. This was a turning point in her recovery.

Take a few moments to reflect on the areas we talked about earlier in relation to our values, such as family and friends, intimate or partner relationships, work and finances, education or personal growth, health and fitness, leisure, the community or environment, and spirituality. Consider activities in these areas that are meaningful to you and make a note of them in your journal. Would it be worthwhile setting some intentions around doing more of them in the journal?

Life is about doing: The key is finding activities you enjoy and find meaningful. Make a note of them in your journal

Another activity that fosters wellbeing is regularly practising **gratitude.** Research has shown that you only need to tap into gratitude once a week to have a positive effect on mood.[30] A couple of useful strategies from this approach include making a list of three good things that have happened in our lives and next to each one writing what the event means to us or says about us; or simply making a list of three things we are grateful for today; for example, a kind word from someone or a gorgeous flower. The journal is the perfect place to do this.

Practise gratitude regularly: Once a week practise gratitude by writing down three good things that have happened, no matter how small.

10. Consider complementary therapies or medication if needed

Complementary therapies are often used and can be of assistance. Massage or herbal medication may be useful to help deal with mental health issues. Various herbal medicines or supplements are used for mild depression and anxiety, such as St John's Wort (hypericum) and SAMe (S-adenosyl methionine).

It is often presumed complementary treatments are fully safe, but there may be potential risks. Herbal medicines or supplements can have side effects and interactions with other medicines, so always discuss their use with a qualified healthcare practitioner before taking any complementary medicines.

There is some evidence for complementary approaches such as light therapy (in depression), or yoga or acupuncture (for anxiety).[31] Many people find massage or reiki very calming too.

A range of pharmaceutical medications is used in treating mental health issues. The decision to consider medication often comes down to how severe the mental health problem is and how much it is impacting your functioning. Usually the talking therapies are utilized first, but sometimes there will be such a lot of suffering that we start to think about whether medication might help.

There is a lot of misinformation about medication. You need reliable and balanced information to be able to make an informed decision. Reputable websites can assist, or a doctor can provide information about the various types of medication, their uses and potential side effects.

There is genetic testing now available to help determine which mental health medications are more suitable for an individual. Remember that medication can improve quality of life, and can be lifesaving at times, such as in severe mental illness.

We are not going to discuss medication in detail, but here are some guidelines:

» When there are very troublesome issues with mental health (e.g. moderate or severe symptoms), there may be a place for medication.

» However, make sure a 'whole person' approach is being taken. In general (unless an illness is severe), we start with information, address lifestyle and self-care, and utilize talking therapies.

» When there are significant symptoms, including suicidal thoughts, help should be urgently sought (see Chapter 7).

» Medication should not be the only treatment. Better long-term outcomes occur when talking therapies are also used.

Let's summarize

This chapter has provided a number of foundational steps to enhance our mental health and wellbeing. These involved raising our awareness and identifying what to focus on; being mindful of our emotions; choosing some intentions or goals; and attending to physical health, lifestyle and self-care.

The other steps included connecting with others, tapping into talking therapies; knowing and using our strengths; exploring self-compassion, meaning and purpose; enjoying meaningful activities and practising gratitude. We also considered the place of complementary therapies or medication.

These foundational steps have been informed by a holistic approach. Having a growth mindset and the importance of neuroplasticity for learning and change was highlighted. Many of the steps involve practical tasks and strategies, which we can work on over time.

Many of the strategies we have looked at in this chapter can play a preventive role for mental health and wellbeing, and they can feel good! And thanks to neuroplasticity and a growth mindset, and sometimes just our pure grit, we are all capable of learning, changing and flourishing.

Here are the keys to mental wellbeing identified in this chapter:

» Reflect on your values.

» To understand more about your emotions, be mindful and connect with how they show up in the body.

» When working with intentions and goals, keep the 'why' in mind, keep things very simple, take small steps and celebrate them.

» Have a regular check-up with a doctor.

» Do a lifestyle review.

» Work with your strengths.

» Reflect on ikigai.

» Life is about doing: find activities that are enjoyable and personally meaningful.

» Regularly practise gratitude.

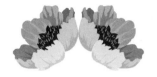

OVERCOMING CHALLENGES AND GROWING MENTAL HEALTH AND WELLBEING

3

Silencing self-criticism
and enhancing self-belief

This chapter tackles a very important issue for women. As explained earlier, we are often trained to look after everyone else ahead of ourselves, and to please others. In addition, we are human and so we naturally compare ourselves to others. This is fostered by media and, in particular, social media.

As a consequence, a common experience is that we are hard on ourselves, may feel like an imposter, or have a strong **inner critic** or self-critical voice in our minds. The thoughts and feelings that this inner critic generates can lead to suffering and a sense of powerlessness. They diminish self-belief and can feel like a heavy door to get past.

Rose struggled with a heavy door, her inner critic.

> An accomplished counsellor and coach, Rose wanted to produce an online course for women learning to be coaches, but struggled with self-doubt. A self-critical voice told her that it would not be 'good enough'. Rose avoided writing the course for a long time, but in the end decided to see a counsellor herself. She identified that the blocks to writing were about wanting it to be 'perfect', for fear that her work would be negatively judged by others. She overcame this fear and worked on her expectations, and wrote the course. It is now online!

In other words, Rose found that she was not powerless and that she had the ability to grow and bring about change. The first step was awareness.

This chapter focuses on understanding how our doors become heavy, and which keys are available to us to open the door to greater self-belief and self-compassion. The aim of fostering greater self-belief and self-compassion is to feel comfortable being our authentic selves and accepting that we are 'enough'. Hopefully after reading and working through this chapter, you will have a greater sense of being enough and the door will start to feel lighter!

The nature of self-belief and origins of the inner critic

Many (or maybe most) women, whether new mothers, older women, women in paid employment, sportswomen or in women in the public eye, report 'low self-esteem' and a struggle with self-doubt. There may be negative self-talk about not being 'good enough' or inadequate in some way. We might recognize these thoughts as coming from a self-critical or disapproving voice in our minds. This voice, which can be mean, attacking or derogatory, is often called the inner critic. It is characterized by thoughts such as, 'I should have done better' or 'what is wrong with me?' We may even talk about 'hating' or loathing ourselves.

I recently read an article in the newspaper about Australian tennis professional, Ash Barty, who'd recently won Wimbledon and retired soon after. The article contains a quote from Barty's new book, where she speaks about her struggles with two inner voices: 'One whispers "Ash you're not good enough"; and the other replies "yes you are — come on Ash." Sometimes one voice would win out over the other.'[1]

It is as though we are programmed to be hard on ourselves, with the inner critic often saying we are not 'good enough'.

Many of the thoughts our inner critic generates can create obstacles to being our authentic or true self, to doing what we want to or value in life, and can cause suffering or loss of power. Self-criticism can contribute to a sense of shame, symptoms of stress and anxiety, and loss of confidence or low mood. The inner critic and the related struggle with self-belief can be like a heavy door to get through.

Before going any further, let's consider some of the commonly used words related to our sense of being 'enough'. This is an important step as there are misconceptions related to some of these terms.

» **Self-esteem** is not a particularly useful term. We tend to think people either have high or low self-esteem or somehow need to get more of it, whatever 'it' is. We might also criticize ourselves for not having enough of 'it'. Self-esteem actually refers to how we view ourselves, often in comparison to others. It describes our opinion of ourselves. It comes from life experiences and relates to our thoughts and beliefs about ourselves.

» We may experience **self-doubt** to a greater or lesser degree. The opposite of self-doubt is having a sense of **self-worth**. Again, this relates to our thoughts about ourselves, and these influence our self-confidence.

» Helpful underlying beliefs about ourselves are referred to as **self-belief**, and these drive our self-talk and confidence.

» **Self-acceptance** refers to accepting that we do well at some things and that we also make mistakes. Sometimes we will mess up or fail, but we can learn from our mistakes or failures.

» Finally, the term **self-compassion** means that we are kind and understanding towards ourselves, instead of criticizing and judging ourselves harshly.[2]

In summary, the most helpful terms seem to be self-belief and self-compassion, and these are the ones used in this book. The good news is that we can grow both of these and feel the benefits.

Remember that we can grow: We can grow both self-compassion and self-belief, the underlying beliefs about ourselves which drive our thoughts.

The development of self-belief

From the moment we are born, there are many influences on our self-belief. We are like sponges growing up, absorbing all the positive and negative messages that we receive from society. Plus, we are human and have a range of life experiences, individual characteristics and personality traits. Our self-belief is shaped by all of these influences, so let's now talk about the main ones.

The society in which we live

We are influenced in positive and negative ways by society. Take a moment to imagine standing under an umbrella, and within this umbrella are all the influences of society, including family, friends, media and the wider community. This also includes the dominant ideas that society holds. As we stand under the umbrella, these influences shape our mind. As a result, we may take on the view that to be worthy we must be attractive, nurturing, smart, popular, successful, able to do it all and even more.

Under all of life's influences, we may take on the view that to be 'worthy' we must have and be able to do it all!

It does not take much to see that achieving these ideals is unrealistic. We might want to match a woman presenting their life as 'perfect' on social media, or exhaust ourselves trying to do everything at the same time. New mothers, for example, may express the desire to be a 'great mother', have a clean house, keep progressing with work, and be a wonderful partner. But we have to consider whether all of this is humanly possible.

We can also be conditioned by these influences to act in ways that ensure they are viewed as 'nice', 'good' or 'likeable'. And we may be shamed when we do something that might be viewed as 'not likeable'. Think about how female politicians have so often been humiliated and shamed about their appearance or actions. Remember that shame goes to our core and is related to thoughts about being a 'bad person', and has the effect of reducing our power.

Shame is related to thoughts about being a 'bad person' and has the effect of reducing our power.

Brené Brown has done a lot of work in the area of shame. She writes about 'the shame web', explaining that women experience shame as a web of layered, conflicting and competing expectations from society. These dictate 'who we should be, what we should be and how we should be!' She speaks about shame being about fear, in particular fear that we will be ridiculed, rejected or deemed unworthy.[3]

Interestingly, the inner critic is sometimes seen as protective, helping us avoid these experiences of shaming and to remain in our 'tribe'. However, the downside to self-criticism very often outweighs the protective aspect. Shame is often followed by self-blaming, which can lead to self-loathing or even blaming others.

Being human

Comparison is hardwired into the brain to help us survive by ascertaining whether we are in danger. For example, if we are wandering down a street and see a group of people carrying weapons, we want to compare ourselves to them and stay safe by running away! Most of the time we are not in danger, but we have a natural tendency to compare ourselves to other people, whether they are known to us or not.

The challenge is that comparison can be a huge trap! This is because what we see of others tends to be just a snapshot of their lives. They generally do not have their worst moments or vulnerabilities on show. For example, on social media, most people don't post pictures of themselves when they first get up in the morning or during some crisis in their lives. They present a story about themselves such as 'I'm successful' or 'perfect' or 'beautiful'. Remember that when we compare, we despair!

Comparison can be a huge trap. Remember that what we see of others tends to be just a snapshot of their lives. They don't show us their worst moments.

In addition, we live in a world in which success is often defined by material possessions, and this can be another comparison trap. As well as managing our natural tendency to compare, we need to deal with advertising. As author Johan Hari explains in his book *Lost Connections*, since the 1920s advertising has aimed to make us think that we are lacking in something and to feel inadequate, and then offers the product as the solution.[4]

Our life experiences

Experiencing a lot of criticism while growing up will impact our thoughts about ourselves. When a child receives unjustified criticism from others, especially from caregivers or authority figures, they can take on the belief that they are not 'good enough' or are not achieving enough. Criticism from others can be internalized as the truth. This is how the inner critic develops.

Ongoing experiences in families, relationships or the workplace continue to influence our self-belief. If we come across a bully or an abusive person, their negative and intimidating behaviours can significantly erode our self-belief and confidence. If we are in a relationship with a partner who is overly critical, has unreasonable expectations or is abusive, this will have the same effect.

Our personality and thinking style

We may be pushed around by different personality traits such as perfectionism. This can particularly impact new mothers, women undertaking studies or those in the workforce. Please read more on this trait in Chapter 6.

Negative thinking about our achievements or ourselves can also impact self-belief, self-confidence and mood. Developing more optimistic thinking can help us focus on positive events in life and our own positive attributes. We will look at ways to do this later in the chapter.

How does low self-belief influence our health and wellbeing?

Low self-belief and self-criticism can affect our health and wellbeing in many ways:

» contributing to stress, anxiety and low mood

» negatively affecting sleep and eating habits, or ability to exercise, and therefore general health

» it can be tiring and distracting to focus on our limitations, and low self-belief can affect coping behaviours, such as not having the energy to engage in leisure activities

» affecting our confidence with others, and possibly preventing us from socializing or going to work functions

» it may affect assertiveness, or cause us to not put ourselves forward for tasks at work through fear of failing.

Because of these impacts it is worthwhile investing in strategies to grow self-belief.

Foster self-belief every day: Positive self-belief is protective for our physical and mental health. Foster it every day.

Increasing our self-belief and silencing the inner critic

Let's now consider a few different ways to increase self-belief and silence that inner critic.

Imagine that there is a table in front of you, with different ideas on the table for you to consider. You can choose the ones that seem to fit you best. The ideas come from various models of therapy or philosophical approaches, and are based on evidence and experience. Most are very practical, as this is often what is needed to bring about change. What we are looking out for is a key (or several) to help open that heavy door!

Here are six ways to silence that inner critic and grow self-belief.

1. Change your thinking

Cognitive Behaviour Therapy is based on the idea that our thoughts, feelings and behaviours all influence each other. That means, for example, that our thoughts influence how we feel and what we do, and vice versa. So, to feel or act more confidently, sometimes we will need to work on our thinking.

In addition, thoughts can reflect our subconscious beliefs about ourselves. It is worth being aware of some of these as they can keep the door to self-belief closed. These are also called 'core' beliefs and Albert Ellis, one of the founders of cognitive based therapies, identified a number.

Core beliefs include: 'I need to be loved and approved of by all significant people in my life' or 'I need to be 100 per cent competent, adequate and achieving in every area of my life'.[5] They may show themselves through a need to prove ourselves to others through our achievements, needing to gain everyone's approval or to be loved to see ourselves as worthwhile.

These beliefs are not all bad, but they are not realistic and may come at a cost. Let's consider some alternatives. Achievements give a sense of satisfaction, but they do not necessarily grow self-belief. Our worth is not about what we achieve. Also, we all seek approval from others, but we have to be careful not to measure our sense of worth based on the praise of others. What is important is what we think about ourselves, and whether we accept ourselves and what we do.

We are not our achievements or how others see us. We are 'enough' just as we are!

Remember that it has taken years for thoughts and underlying beliefs to be shaped, so it will take some time and practice to change them.

There is a series of steps involved in identifying our thoughts, recognizing any traps in our thinking and learning to challenge them. These will be covered in detail in Chapter 4, and we will look more into core beliefs in Chapter 6. The key is being less harsh on ourselves, and using kinder self-talk.

In relation to self-belief in particular, it can be useful to make some notes about your strengths and what you see as any 'weaknesses', such as 'I am hopeless in social situations'. Then take some time to reassess and be a bit gentler with yourself. The aim is to reframe and be less harsh, for example: 'I tend to be quiet in social situations. I am working on having the confidence to say what I choose to.'

We have over 60,000 thoughts a day, because our brain is constantly processing what is going on around us and generating thoughts. The problem is that we can become 'fused' or hooked by any of our thoughts, even the many untrue ones. Thoughts such as 'I'll fail' or 'I don't have what it takes' can give us a reason not to do something and our mind can put obstacles in our way or predict poor outcomes.[6]

Another way of dealing with unhelpful thoughts comes from **Acceptance and Commitment Therapy**. Called **defusion**, it takes the power out of thoughts. Defusion involves noticing our thoughts, stepping back from them and holding them more lightly. We can then choose whether to pay attention to them or let them pass. In other words, defusion helps us realize that a thought is just a thought! Please see Chapter 4 for more on this therapy.

2. Change our stories

We understand the world and ourselves through narratives or stories, and this is the basis of **Narrative Therapy**. We have many stories about ourselves; some are positive and others negative. These stories are made up of events that are linked together across time in a way that makes sense to us. In fact, we develop many stories about our lives.

Stories may be about our abilities, our struggles, our work, dreams or relationships. These have been developed under the influence of dominant ideas in society, for example, what an ideal woman looks like or what an ideal mother does.

When we are being pushed around by a self-critical story, it can seem as though all we are is the story. However, this is not the case. Just recognizing this can help us get some separation from the story.

There will always be exceptions to the dominant story. Just like panning for gold, we need to look for the flecks of gold, or the exceptions, amongst the dust. In this way we can start to build up an 'alternate story', which might include the times we got through a difficult situation, made progress or achieved something, no matter how small.

Change your self-critical stories: We all have stories about ourselves, and some dominate our lives. We need to explore these, see them for what they are, and gradually build up an alternative story.

We have our strengths and have survived many challenges, and we can work on incorporating strengths into our stories. For example, even though we may have experienced rejection in life, in spite of this we still make our way through life and make meaningful connections. We will talk more about the narrative approach in Chapters 4 and 6.

3. Explore acceptance

We live in a world where some things are within our control, and many are out of our control. The challenge is to accept what is out of our control and focus on what we can do in relation to things we can control to help create a meaningful life.[7]

Acceptance is a powerful concept in life. This is one of the most challenging things to do, as life involves good as well as bad events. Equally, feelings are sometimes wonderful and at other times awful. **Acceptance** is about our willingness to experience the whole range of feelings, without trying to change them. One approach is to become less caught up in painful feelings or thoughts, including the self-critical ones, and be more involved in doing what we care about and value.

4. Practise mindfulness

As mentioned earlier, mindfulness involves paying attention on purpose, to experience the present moment, as opposed to being caught up in thoughts or feelings. It also means being non-judgmental about what we are experiencing. When having a cup of coffee in the sunshine, for example, pay attention to the taste and smell of the coffee and the warmth of the sun, rather than getting caught up with worries or thoughts.

In the same way, we can be mindful of our thoughts and feelings, noticing them, rather than getting caught up with them. Through mindfulness we can learn that thoughts and feelings come and go. In this way mindfulness can also assist us to develop greater self-acceptance, as we experience less judgment about ourselves.

5. Focus on positive emotions and accomplishment

As outlined in Chapter 2, Positive Psychology focuses on human strengths and psychological wellbeing. It encourages us to know our strengths and to use them more. Research has found that if we know and use our abilities and strengths, we will be happier and more confident.

This approach has also found that enhancing relationships, finding meaning in life through our passions and a sense of purpose, and having a sense of accomplishment can enhance our self-confidence and wellbeing.

It also suggests visualization as a useful strategy for self-confidence. Athletes use this strategy to focus before their events. They visualize their performance and a successful outcome, and this has been shown to help. Consider using visualization before an interaction or event. To do this, make yourself comfortable, close your eyes and imagine the event occurring in positive way with a satisfactory outcome.

6. Other tips for self-belief

A range of approaches and strategies have been put on the table already. But there are some more tips to help in enhancing self-belief. Take a few moments to look through them and see if any of these might assist:

» Continue to develop self-awareness through noticing your mood and thoughts, perhaps making notes in the journal. Read books, watch films or documentaries or talk with others. Explore meditation, reflection or prayer. What about doing some personal development courses or further studies?

» Act like the person you want to be! A colleague once said that when she feels low and lacking in self-worth, she focuses on what it is like to be feeling better in herself and more confident. This gets her back to feeling more positive. Tapping into a memory of a time associated with good feelings can also help. Sometimes 'faking it until you make it' in relation to self-confidence can also assist.

>> We can change how we feel by doing the opposite with our posture and facial expression. It is time to stand tall and smile!

>> Enjoy positive quotes, such as Theodore Roosevelt's 'Believe you can and you're halfway there.'

>> Accept compliments; simply say thank you!

>> And don't forget to celebrate successes. Maybe take some time out, share success with a friend, or enjoy a reward to acknowledge the success.

Do the opposite: It can help to act like the person we want to be. Stand tall and smile!

A focus on self-compassion

Most of us have grown up with the golden rule, 'Treat others as you would like others to treat you.' With compassion for others, we are aware of their suffering and feel moved by it. We feel empathy, caring and the desire to help. Having self-compassion is just like having compassion for others. It means we are kind and understanding towards ourselves when faced by our personal challenges, instead of judging harshly.[8]

Self-compassion means we are kind and understanding towards ourselves, instead of being self-critical.

Developing greater self-compassion is a golden key to being less self-critical and growing our self-belief. Having compassion means we offer kindness to others when they make mistakes. When we feel compassion for another person, we are recognizing that suffering and imperfection are part of being human. And self-compassion involves acting the same way towards ourselves when we are having a difficult time.

Engaging in random acts of kindness, such as helping someone in need, can lead to feeling more connected with others and more positive within ourselves. Self-compassion has been shown to be associated with happiness, optimism, wisdom, curiosity and emotional intelligence. It can also help in dealing with pain and help our relationships.[9] One of the reasons self-compassion can do all of this is that it activates the soothing and calming parts of our nervous system (parasympathetic and ventral vagal system, outlined in Chapter 2).[10] Understanding this beneficial effect of self-compassion may encourage us to see it not only as part of our daily wellbeing, but also as a powerful strategy to help us achieve our potential and flourish.

Skills related to self-compassion

Humans have an innate capacity to be caring and compassionate, but sometimes having experiences that create humiliation or shame, and being taught that it is not okay to be kind to ourselves when growing up can lead to resistance to self-compassion as an adult.

Psychologist and author Stan Steidl writes about the importance of overcoming any blocks to receiving or giving compassion. One place to begin is by being aware of potential blocks to compassion such as thinking compassion will lead to a sense of weakness or vulnerability, or that self-compassion is self-indulgent. We may then choose to work through these blocks ourselves or seek out a therapist.

Learning some ways to soothe emotions can assist in this process (see Chapter 7). Calm breathing is useful, and we can even breathe compassionately by placing our hands over our heart as a gesture of kindness and comfort towards ourselves. This is worth trying, as it feels very good!

Steidl also writes that self-compassion involves courage, wisdom and commitment to wellbeing. He describes it as a particular version of ourselves and says that we can get to know that part better and gradually strengthen it over time. Remember that there is no rush, as learning new approaches and behaviours takes time.[11]

Self-compassion takes time: There is no rush with self-compassion or kindness. Remember that learning a new way of being takes time and practice.

If shame is having an influence on you, it is important to work through this and get to better know your authentic self. Brené Brown speaks about developing 'shame resilience' over time, and how empathy is a strong antidote to shame.[12] As mentioned earlier, empathy is about being able to tap into your own experiences in order to connect with an experience someone is relating to you, or being able to see it from their perspective. When we are non-judgmental with ourselves, we experience greater empathy and compassion for ourselves.

It is also about connection with others in our support networks or establishing more support. Our supports give us comfort and a sense of power. Empathy is also about our relationship with ourselves. We spend more time with ourselves than anyone else! This relationship is very important, and we need to practise empathy with ourselves.

Revisit the discussion in the first part of this chapter about the trap of comparison and remember that you are human! Aim to drop unhelpful comparisons and to tackle self-criticism. You can also bring some compassion to the inner critic by removing any harsh words and using kinder words in your self-talk.

And remember that what we might perceive as a 'weakness' can also be a strength. An example is being more sensitive than we might like. This could be seen as a weakness, but it also means we are more sensitive to the needs of others. Or being stubborn may also mean we are very determined and don't give up. It might be helpful to reflect on any perceived weaknesses in your journal and see if there is a strength hidden there!

Sometimes perceived weaknesses are also strengths: It is important to recognize that our perceived weaknesses might have a flipside that is actually a strength in life.

The loving-kindness meditation

A good way to remind yourself to practise self-compassion is through the 'loving-kindness' meditation, which is based on a poem from Buddhism: 'May I be filled with loving-kindness, may I be well, may I be peaceful and at ease, may I be happy.' The loving-kindness meditation puts you in touch with warm and compassionate feelings in an openhearted way, and directs these feelings to yourself and then to others.[13] Here is a script for the meditation.

Make yourself comfortable and let your eyes close. Focus your attention on your breath and relax a little more with each breath out. Relax your body from the top of your head down to the tips of your toes. Then focus on the region of your heart. Get in touch with your heart, and reflect on a person for whom you feel warm, tender and compassionate feelings. This could be a child, partner or a pet. Imagine yourself with this loved one and notice how you feel. Extend loving-kindness to them by saying in your mind, 'May you be well, may you be at ease, may you be happy and at peace.'

Hold onto the warm and compassionate feelings. And now extend that warmth to yourself. Extend kindness to yourself as you do others, and allow your heart to radiate with love.

When you are ready, radiate your warm and compassionate feelings to others: first to a person you know well, and then call to mind others with whom you have connections. Ultimately, you can extend loving-kindness to all if you choose.

When you are ready, open your eyes and come back to the here and now.

You can be creative with self-compassion, such as expressing compassion towards yourself through art or writing. For example, write a letter to yourself expressing understanding, empathy and validation in relation to challenges, focusing on your strengths, and giving some reassurance, encouragement and support.[14] This might be something else for the journal.

Other activities that can foster self-compassion include helping family, volunteering, calling a friend to see how they are doing, smiling at someone, animal rescue, donating unused items to charity, writing a thank you note, expressing how you feel to someone you trust, finding time to read a book or watch a movie or cooking a favourite meal for yourself.[15]

Time to reflect: As you develop self-compassion, reflect in your journal on the ways you will act differently and treat others and yourself differently.[16]

 ## Let's summarize

In this very important chapter, we have explored the nature of self-belief and the origins of the inner critic. This critic can grow very loud and can get in the way of thinking, feeling and doing as we wish.

We looked at how self-belief is influenced by society, by being human and naturally comparing ourselves to others, and by our life experiences. Our personality and thinking style (whether more optimistic or pessimistic) also play a role.

Low self-belief and self-criticism can adversely affect our mental health and wellbeing, so it is very important to work on growing self-belief. We can do this by changing our thinking patterns and some of our stories about ourselves. Mindfulness again was highlighted as having a role in building self-belief by helping us become more self-aware and less judgmental.

Self-compassion was one of the most important keys to lightening the heavy door of self-criticism. Through self-compassion, we can learn to soothe our emotions, connect with others and reframe perceived 'weaknesses' as strengths!

As our main relationship in life is with ourselves, it is a good investment to work on this relationship. Write down any useful keys in the journal. As we learn to be kinder to ourselves, we will discover our authentic and flourishing selves.

Here is a reminder about the keys to growing our self-belief:

» Remember that we can grow.

» Foster self-belief every day.

» Change self-critical stories.

» Do the opposite: Act like the person you want to be.

» Self-compassion takes time.

» Sometimes weaknesses are also strengths.

» Take time to reflect.

4

Taming stress and anxiety

"

Nothing is so much to be feared as fear.

— Henry David Thoreau

Stress is part of everyday life, and anxiety is there to protect us. But high levels of stress or anxiety can feel frightening and awful, and be very hard to manage. It can be difficult to untangle what might be causing anxiety and how to manage it. Sometimes there might not be a clear cause, and at other times it is evident that work stressors, interpersonal issues or past trauma are triggers.

In this chapter we will cover quite a lot of territory, including more information about several therapies. This information will be relevant to later chapters as well. Please try out the keys and strategies outlined. The more you understand and the more keys you hold, the less influence stress and anxiety will exert in your life, and the more content and empowered you will feel.

Many of the strategies in this chapter are useful to know about for our day-to-day lives, whether or not we are being pushed around by stress or anxiety. Strategies such as mindfulness and meditation can aid our sense of mental (and physical) wellbeing when incorporated into our lives. So please read on, make a few notes in your journal, and adopt any of the ideas that might help with flourishing!

Some definitions

Stress comes from demands on us, whether related to earning money, finding time to get to the gym, or meeting the needs of partners or family. **Anxiety** is a normal feeling. It is related to fear, and it may arise in situations that are very stressful, or where there is some perceived 'threat', such as saying no to someone or attending a job interview. We can also feel **overwhelmed** or overcome with emotion when there is a lot to deal with and it all seems too much to handle.

The nature of stress and anxiety

A reasonable level of stress (called **eustress**) can help us get things accomplished, and we often perform better when there is some stress. However, we will feel uncomfortably stressed when we see demands as being beyond our ability to cope, especially when involving a situation that is unpredictable or we don't have a lot of control. Our bodies and minds are designed to respond to sudden or short-term stress. However, a lot of today's stresses are more chronic or ongoing.

Anxiety is a response to threat or danger, and it helps us to survive. We have an in-built stress response, which is an automatic response by our nervous system to protect us, and certain chemicals in the body (brain cell messengers or neurotransmitters and hormones) are involved when there is anxiety. We will look at the stress response in a short while.

Anxiety can be very distressing and can trigger more fear, and interfere greatly with life. It can lead us to avoid doing many things; for example, if anxiety is experienced while driving on a freeway, we might avoid going on freeways, or if anxiety occurs in work meetings, we may try to avoid them. Anxiety is often about something that might happen in the future, such as feeling anxious before giving a talk or taking a driving test.

Anxiety is often future-based and can lead to avoidance of things we fear.

We can recognize anxiety by what we experience in the body and mind, such as racing thoughts, a feeling of dread, sweating, muscle tension, palpitations (the heart beating fast in the chest) or changes to breathing (often becoming fast and shallow). Other symptoms include headaches, feeling irritable or angry, finding it hard to get to sleep, having broken sleep or having a lowered sex drive.

Experiencing stress or anxiety is different from having an anxiety disorder. When anxiety is severe or persists and impacts our ability to do what we need and want to do, it might fit with being called a disorder. Worldwide, anxiety disorders are among the most common mental health disorders. Our thinking about the different forms of anxiety is returning to the concept that an individual may have a vulnerability to anxiety and may experience different forms of it over time.

Understanding the currently used names and features of anxiety disorders may be useful. Some key ones are:

» phobias or specific fears; for example, a fear of heights or snakes

» social anxiety, which is based on a fear of embarrassment in social situations or being thought of negatively by others

» panic disorder, involving 'panic attacks' or repeated episodes of severe anxiety

» agoraphobia or a fear of not being able to escape or of open spaces, and may or may not occur with panic disorder

» generalized anxiety or worrying most of the time about a range of issues.

There are a few other related disorders to be aware of. Obsessive-compulsive disorder involves repeatedly thinking about things that might be harmful to oneself or others, and possibly carrying out repeated behaviours to relieve that worry, such as checking or cleaning (compulsions). Post-traumatic stress disorder, which can follow traumatic events, has specific features such as nightmares or flashbacks, and can trigger anxiety symptoms and avoidance. Anxiety related to having a severe illness has become more of a problem during the COVID-19 pandemic. We will look at this issue later in this chapter.

The causes of stress and anxiety

We can feel stress in response to any demand or perceived threat we face (such as losing a job). Chronic stress is often experienced in our day-to-day modern lives, with family, financial or work stressors.

Technology has added many layers of stress, including keeping up to date with developments, the ever-present texts, alerts and emails (and the expectations about responding quickly), and managing social media.

We know that various factors can play a role in causing or worsening stress or anxiety. Some families are more prone to anxiety. Health issues such as chronic illness or pain, or hormonal changes such as premenstrual, postnatal or menopausal changes, may contribute (more on this in Chapter 8). Some medications may trigger anxiety (e.g. methamphetamines, some antidepressants initially when used, caffeine or energy drinks).

The level of stress and anxiety also depends on the type and number of life stressors, whether related to family pressures, living conditions or relationships. In relation to work, high demands, poor support or challenging relationships with co-workers can be stressful. Juggling multiple roles and responsibilities in life or trying to be everything to everyone will also be highly stressful.

Some people have personality traits that can contribute to stress and anxiety, such as being a perfectionist (see Chapter 6). How we think can also influence anxiety. Being more pessimistic may trigger more anxiety or wanting to always feel in control of things. The level of anxiety can also relate to coping skills, for example being able to problem-solve can reduce worry, or recognizing the need to relax regularly.

Upbringing and how we 'attach' to our parents or caregivers can also play a role (more on this in Chapter 9). Children may learn to be anxious in a particular situation, which is more likely if there is neglect or abuse. An underlying fear of abandonment or rejection can be retriggered later in life. And trauma such as accidents, bullying and violence can result in anxiety.

Social disadvantage can contribute to experiencing anxiety, as can social isolation. Loneliness has been found to have very significant impacts on our physical and emotional health and wellbeing, and as a result some countries have government ministers for loneliness. Spiritual triggers to stress and anxiety can also occur, such as issues within a church, or personal struggles with beliefs.

There are many causes of anxiety, ranging from our genetics to our upbringing, our learning, personality traits, social disadvantage or trauma.

When we see a therapist, they will explore our stories, listening out for possible causes or triggers for anxiety. Sometimes these will be clear, and at other times not so clear. Symptoms of social anxiety often arise in adolescence when peers are so important to young people. Panic episodes are often seen in early adulthood, and there may or may not be a particular stress or trauma at the time, or a family history of panic. Generalized anxiety is often present from childhood, and there may be other family members experiencing anxiety. It may worsen at times of stress.

How the mind and body respond to stress and anxiety

We respond to threat with the 'fight, flight or freeze' or stress response. This response is there to protect us and dates to prehistoric times. Thousands of years ago, when out hunting for food, humans might have come face to face with a dangerous animal. We saw the animal, our brain recognized the danger, then a number of changes happened in the body to prepare us to fight the animal, run back to the cave or freeze ('play dead').

This response is still automatic in our brains today. The limbic brain, along with other parts of the brain (hypothalamus) and body, are responsible for this response. They communicate with and activate the 'autonomic' or automatic part of the nervous system, especially the 'sympathetic' arm of it (see p. 47).

The fight or flight response also involves the release of a number of stress hormones, including adrenaline. This results in a faster heart rate, to pump blood to the muscles so we can run or fight. Less blood goes to the brain, the skin, the fingers and toes and the gut. We don't need to think or digest food if we are about to be eaten! This is why we may feel foggy, tingly or nauseated when stressed.

Glucose moves into the bloodstream to provide energy, and we become more alert through the senses (hearing, sight, smell). We sweat more to cool the body, and the breathing rate can become quicker and shallower to get more oxygen around the body. We can feel light-headed as a result of the increased breathing rate.

These changes in the body generally won't harm us, but they don't feel good. They don't mean that we are 'losing it'. Remember that in the modern world, the threat may no longer be a wild animal, but it could be an upsetting social media post, a job loss or conflict. In the modern world there may be many threats at the same time, and stress may become chronic in nature.

> Changes in the body and brain related to stress don't feel good, but they won't harm us. And they don't mean that we are 'losing it'.

In addition, in response to threat we may 'fawn' and 'flock'. We see fawning behaviours in situations where there is a power difference, for example, in some workplaces or when there is intimate partner violence. The person who is fawning becomes agreeable or submissive basically to survive. The flock response refers to seeking out like individuals for support.

Ways to deal with stress and anxiety

Let's look at a few helpful steps to assist with anxiety, plus a few extra strategies. See what seems a good fit for you, and maybe jot down some of the ideas in your journal.

We are going to explore five steps in particular:

1. Review lifestyle and have a check-up.
2. Reduce your 'stress bucket' and learn to relax.
3. Identify and work through related issues.
4. Tap into talking therapies.

5. Utlilize self-help, and consider complementary therapies or medication.

1. Review lifestyle and have a check-up

Focusing on a healthy lifestyle is always important in reducing stress and anxiety. In particular, limiting alcohol and caffeine, getting some regular exercise, eating healthily, improving sleep, managing stress, taking time out to relax, reducing substance-use, enjoying activities and connecting with others can all help.

Practising mindfulness regularly, and disconnecting at times from phones, tablets or laptops can also assist. And don't forget about humour — having a good laugh can help relieve stress and anxiety.

Have a check-up to make sure the symptoms of physical illnesses such as anaemia or an overactive thyroid are not mimicking anxiety. This is vital and is illustrated by the story of Wendy.

> Wendy began to cry as soon as she entered the doctor's room, saying that she felt really anxious. The doctor then noticed that her eyes looked prominent, and found that her pulse was racing. Wendy had hyperthyroidism that had triggered her symptoms. Once treated, she felt a lot better.

Apart from helping sort out physical health issues, a doctor can also listen and offer support, discuss lifestyle and provide information. They can assist in developing a plan of management, including what to do in a crisis. Some are trained in particular therapies, and they can also suggest an appropriate therapist.

2. Reduce your 'stress bucket' and learn to relax

Each day is filled with demands, from getting up in the morning, to doing things for family members, going to work and paying bills. Imagine that we all have a bucket inside of us! The bucket can hold a certain amount of stress or anxiety, but each demand adds more to the bucket and it gradually fills up.

If the bucket gets too full, we might find that when a final stressful event happens (even a very small thing), we can feel overwhelmed and our stress level 'spills over' with feelings like irritability or frustration, or out-of-character behaviours. We might cry or become angry, for example, in response to something minor happening. This is a good indication that your stress level needs to be lowered.

The opposite of feeling stressed or anxious is feeling relaxed — so learning how to relax is vital. There are different ways to relax and these generally work via the 'parasympathetic' arm of the nervous system (including the vagus nerve). The easiest way to activate this system and to relax is to breathe effectively. When we feel calm we take about twelve breaths per minute; when anxious this might rise to 25. This is why relaxation strategies so often involve breathing.

Here are a few examples of breathing techniques to try out:

» Sit or stand up straight. Place your right hand on your upper chest and your left on your abdomen; take medium-sized breaths, focusing on breathing down into the belly. Feel the abdomen move in as you breathe out and out as you breathe in. Aim to breathe in for three counts and out for three counts — counting in, two, three and out, two, three — and this will lead to about ten breaths a minute.

» Some people use 4-7-8 breathing, which involves breathing in for 4 seconds, holding the breath for 7 seconds and breathing out for 8 seconds.

» If this is uncomfortable, try box breathing. Imagine a square shape and follow each side in your mind. Travel up the left-hand side as you breathe in slowly for four counts, across the top as you hold your breath for four counts, down the right hand side as you breathe out for four counts, then hold for four across the bottom and back to the start for four counts. Keep repeating these steps.

» Find a piece of paper and a pen. Place your hand on the paper and slowly draw around your thumb, breathing in with the upstroke, and out with the downstroke. Repeat with each finger.

Physical relaxation is another great relaxation strategy. Progressive muscle relaxation focuses on different muscle groups from head to toe, letting go of any tension in each area. Other relaxation techniques include imagining a pleasant and safe place, such as a garden or a beach. Various forms of meditation may be used. These focus our attention and often incorporate breathing techniques.

Use breathing or relaxation techniques: Experiment with breathing and relaxation strategies. It may be easier to be guided via a recording or app. Many are now available, such as Smiling Mind.

Whichever relaxation strategies you use, aim to do them regularly. For example, even a few minutes of meditation each day can be helpful. Fifteen to 20 minutes is even better! By doing this, your anxiety will lessen over time. Some women prefer to tap into activities such as physical exercise, massage, yoga, music or being creative to relax. The important thing is to spend some time relaxing and emptying the stress bucket!

Related techniques are called grounding techniques. These can be used to reduce anxiety symptoms, especially when they are overwhelming and our nervous systems are in a state of 'hyperarousal' (if we are very anxious and vigilant). The breathing techniques mentioned above, especially 4-7-8 breathing, can help ground us, or we can pay attention to what is around us, such as our feet on the floor and hands on our laps, and how they feel, letting our body be supported by the chair and noticing the feeling of gravity pushing down through our body.

The 5-4-3-2-1 exercise or 'noticing five things' can also help. This involves noticing five things we can see, four things we can hear, three things we can feel (such as the seat we are sitting on), two things we can smell, one thing we can taste. If this is too much to remember, it can be simplified to three things you can see, two things you can feel, and one thing you can hear.

Grounding can be useful: Try grounding when overwhelmed, such as breathing strategies or 'noticing five things'.

There is a series of other activities to stimulate the parasympathetic nervous system (ventral vagus nerve) called 'vagus hacks'. These produce a feeling of calm and include breathing techniques, singing, humming, exercise and cold water (swimming, splashing on face). When we go out into nature and look into the distance (out to sea, or to distant hills) this calming response is also activated.

Sometimes other strategies are needed to reduce the level of stress in the bucket. These might include getting more sleep, or possibly learning to say no more often, delegating or dropping some tasks, and setting boundaries with others. We will look at boundary setting in Chapter 7. And the strategies in the next section about dealing with causes of stress may also help reduce the level in our bucket.

3. Identify and work through related issues

It can help to identify the issues causing stress and anxiety, and actually write them down in your journal to get them out of your head and onto paper. There may be external causes, such as work, relationship problems or financial stress; or internal ones, such as demands or expectations we might place on ourselves.

We may be impacted by high expectations we put on ourselves, for example to look or behave in certain ways, or in relation to being a mother or caring for a family. Equally, some troublesome underlying beliefs about others, the world or us can trigger anxious thoughts. We spoke about some of these 'core beliefs' in Chapter 3. They are formed while growing up and can feed anxiety. We may not even be aware that they are there and influencing our thinking.

We have mentioned a couple of common core beliefs previously, such as, 'I must always be competent or approved of'. Others in anxiety are 'I must be 100 per cent in control at all times' and 'My life should progress smoothly'. The thoughts that stem from these beliefs may sound like, 'I'm never good enough' or 'I'm hopeless'. Remember that these thoughts are not based on truth and can be challenged! We will look into other ways of dealing with core beliefs in Chapter 6.

Author Stephen Covey wrote about the 'circle of influence'. This refers to two circles, one being the circle of concern, which contains factors outside of our control, such as the weather or traffic, and the other being the circle of influence which houses factors that we can control, such as what we do and say, and how we care for ourselves. When we spend time and energy on the circle of concern, we can feel low in mood and helpless, and when we focus more on the circle of influence, we feel more positive and uplifted, and we have a greater sense of agency or ability to influence things.[1]

A related strategy involves 'three boxes in life'. The first box represents us, including our goals and interests; the second represents other people; and the third the world we live in (politics, society, environment). We can lift the lid on the first and take a look inside at any time, and we can spend a lot of time dealing with what's in it and have a lot of influence over it. With the second, we can help or hinder others, but only influence it to a limited degree. With the third, we can run for politics or plant trees, but again, there are limits to what we can do.

There are things within our control and many things outside of our control. We need to concentrate on what we can actually influence.

Let's remember that two of the main causes of stress in life are **relationship and financial issues**. Relationship stress will be dealt with in Chapter 9, but we will consider financial stress here. Many people live with severe financial stress, which can lead to anxiety or overwhelm. It can also trigger health problems. There can be many causes of financial stress, related to limited earnings and rising living costs. The cost of housing is also a major issue for women.

Seeking financial assistance and advice may assist, and some counsellors deal specifically with this area. Setting some goals or using problem-solving may help, such as avoiding 'pay afterwards' options, or reducing debt by gradually paying off a credit card. There are also apps to track spending and plan a budget.

A related issue, and one we have already considered, is advertising. This can be a driver to spend money we don't actually have. We are trained in our consumer society to feel a sense of scarcity or that there is 'never enough', or we can experience FOMO (fear of missing out), and that purchasing lots of things will overcome this and also lead to happiness.

The other aspect to our purchases is that they can trigger the release of the chemical messenger dopamine in the brain. We can get a sense of happiness or a 'high' as a result, and so we may 'self-soothe' anxiety or low mood with shopping. This is more of an issue with easy access to online shopping, and the 'high' may be short-lived once we realize how much money has been spent.

Problem-solving can help us deal with some of the issues triggering anxiety. We often have to deal with problems, but like anything else, we might be able to learn something extra to help. Problem-solving is especially useful when anxious feelings feel overwhelming. It involves sorting out what the specific problems are and looking at practical ways to manage them. It helps us to decide on the best possible solution for the problem (not necessarily the most perfect one).

When problem-solving, start with the simpler problems rather than the complex ones. Work through problems one at a time and go through each step one at a time, too. The steps involved in problem-solving are:

» Define the problem in specific yet everyday terms. Spend time really thinking about this. An example of a problem might be: 'I feel stuck in my job and I want to make a change, but I am worried about not having enough money.'

» Make a list of all the possible solutions. Brainstorm as many solutions as possible, even some wild ones (these can always be discarded).

» Think about the pros and cons of each solution.

» Then choose the best possible solution!

Work with problem-solving: This involves working out what the problems are and working through potential solutions step-by-step.

In problem-solving, we also need to predict challenges that might arise and think about how to deal with them. We need a plan for carrying out the solution, which is broken down into small steps. We need to be realistic about whether there are time and resources to carry it through, and we need to review how things are going. Remember that even a partial success is a win, and that we may not resolve the problem with the first solution.

4. Tap into talking therapies

Talking with someone who listens can help us sort through feelings of stress or anxiety. We feel supported, and as we talk, the brain is processing what has happened and we are sorting out a way forward in our own mind. Central to this process is a trusting relationship with a therapist. They will have been trained in a range of different approaches, and there will be variation as to which ones they use in practice. It can be helpful to check this out with them.

Modifying thoughts and actions can change the way we feel. **Cognitive Behaviour Therapy** was introduced in Chapter 3 and is based on the idea that our thoughts, feelings and behaviours all influence each other. For example, what we think and do affects how we feel. Many women come to therapy wanting to change how they feel. We can't change how we feel on the spot, but we can change our feelings by working with thoughts and actions. This is why the therapy incorporates the terms 'cognitive' (thoughts) and 'behavioural'.

So how can this therapy help to reduce anxiety? Let's look for an answer, starting with actions. Examples of actions we can take to reduce anxiety include relaxation techniques. Doing enjoyable activities, such as reading a book or walking, can help us find calm too. Writing down worries in the journal or on a computer, and then putting the book or file away can put the worries away too. Or allocate 'worry time' each day, say 20 minutes, and work on not being hooked back into worry at any other time.

Worry time: Allocate some 'worry time' each day, when worry is the focus. Put worry aside at other times!

We know that anxiety commonly leads to **avoidance**. Examples include avoiding driving a car after an accident or after having a panic attack while driving.

Annabelle was driving on a freeway with her children in the back seat when another car cut in front of her. She had to swerve to avoid a collision. A first panic episode resulted, and after that she avoided driving on the freeway, but this became a practical problem. Therapy helped Annabelle utilize strategies that worked to relieve the anxiety, so that she no longer avoided certain roads.

Avoidance relieves anxiety in the short term, but often causes more distress in the long term. Not all avoidance is negative, but the main thing is that we recognize when it is becoming unhelpful, for example, when it is preventing us from doing things we want or need to do.

Gradual exposure is a therapeutic strategy used to help overcome avoidance. The technique works on the idea that the brain might need to re-learn not be fearful. Exposure involves facing the fear in a gentle way, with small steps. For example, if someone is fearful of going in an elevator, exposure might involve first looking at pictures of elevators, then standing outside an elevator, then being inside the elevator, then going up one floor and then gradually more.

It is important to learn strategies to manage emotional symptoms prior to doing the exposure, such as breathing or grounding techniques, and problem-solving. And if avoidance is a significant issue, consider getting some help from a therapist.

Equally, if experiencing symptoms of any of the disorders mentioned earlier, such as obsessive-compulsive disorder, post-traumatic stress or illness anxiety disorders, it is best to consult with a therapist, as more specialised treatment techniques involving exposure may be needed.

Avoid avoidance and use exposure: Anxiety often tricks us into avoiding situations in which we might feel anxious. Using gradual exposure, or facing the fear via small steps, can help.

We can also work with anxious thoughts to help reduce anxious feelings. We have thousands of thoughts occurring every day quite automatically in our minds. They give us plenty of information, but many are untrue and we don't have to believe them all! There are a number of potential traps in our thinking and we all experience some (or many) or them!

Here are some of the common thinking traps:

» *Black-and-white thinking*: With this thinking style there is no middle ground. For example, if one or two things don't work out for us, we think 'everything' is going wrong.

» *Jumping to conclusions*: This is about making a negative interpretation of things. For example, we might think that someone is thinking negatively about us when there is no evidence of this (called 'mind-reading'); or we might jump to negative conclusions about the future ('crystal-balling').

» *Catastrophizing*: This is overemphasizing the importance of events, so that a small mistake might be perceived as a disaster.

» *Disqualifying the positives*: Discounting any positive experiences and maintaining a negative outlook.

» *'Should' statements*: We speak to ourselves with 'shoulds' and 'musts'. This is often related to setting high expectations, but the emotional result can be guilt or frustration.

» *Labelling*: Applying labels such as 'I'm a loser' or 'I'm a failure'.

We have about 60,000 thousand thoughts a day! Many of them are not true. They are there to give us information, but we don't have to believe them all.

So what do we actually do with our thoughts to change how we feel? Cognitive Behaviour Therapy teaches us to notice our thoughts, to challenge unhelpful or negative ones and to come up with a more helpful thought. This process is often called **reframing**. We may adopt a more positive thought, although the reframed thought doesn't have to be highly positive. The important thing is that it is more balanced or realistic.

There is a series of step to be aware of, and once these are understood and practised, they become second nature and a powerful strategy to reduce anxious feelings. The steps are:

1. Notice and name the feeling (such as sad, anxious or angry).

2. Notice the thoughts. What is the self-talk? (e.g. 'I should be able to do this.')

3. Learn about potential thinking traps (such as black-and-white thinking or crystal-balling), and work on identifying them.

4. Challenge the thoughts (e.g. 'What would I say to a friend if they were having that thought?' 'Don't "should" on myself!')

5. Develop more helpful thoughts by reframing them (e.g. 'Maybe I can do some practice and give it a go.').

Use cognitive strategies to tame anxiety: Be aware of self-talk, watch out for thinking traps, challenge them and come up with more helpful or balanced thoughts.

With anxiety in particular, pay attention to any self-talk that begins with the words, 'What if?' Some of them are useful, such as: 'What if I don't pay my phone bill?' But most are usually future-based and related to worry, such as 'what if' this bad thing happens or the good thing doesn't happen? Consider taking a 'what if' thought, apply the steps above (write them down in the journal) and see how your feelings towards the 'what if' thought changes.

Managing panic episodes

Let's bring this discussion together by looking at panic episodes, in which the fight or flight response goes into overdrive. The symptoms of panic episodes often occur in 'cascades', which means that one symptom follows another, such as feeling breathless being followed by palpitations, then by dizziness. We tend to spiral down, especially with our thinking, having thoughts such as, 'Oh no, it's happening again ... it's getting worse ... it might be my heart ... what if I have a heart attack?'

To interrupt the physical symptoms of anxiety we can use a breathing technique or 'grounding' strategies. These bring attention to the moment and to the senses, rather than getting stuck in the cascade. Examples of grounding techniques are the 5-4-3-2-1 exercise (see p. 93) or doing some stretches.

The AWARE technique may also assist with panic episodes or anxiety. This involves:

» Accept what is going on and acknowledge any symptoms.

» Watch what is going on. Score anxiety on a scale of 1 to 10 (10 the most severe) and breathe.

» Act normally and keep going if need be. Imagine being calm. Take action and use skills such as breathing or grounding to reduce anxiety.

» **R**epeat A-W-A and mentally rehearse being calm and collected.

» **E**xpect the best. Find a way forward that fits with what is important to you.[2]

And to interrupt panicky thinking, you can replace anxious thoughts with calming thoughts. It can useful to carry a 'taming panic' card with some calming thought prompts.

Carry a 'taming panic' card: Make up a card to carry in your wallet or phone. It might say something like this — 'I know what it is: it's anxiety. I will be fine. Breathe and it will pass.'

Let's come back to the freeze response, in which we may feel that we can't move, time seems to stand still, or we feel dissociated or out of touch with our bodies or the situation. Breathing techniques may not be as helpful with this response, but the grounding techniques often are. It may also help to find a place that feels safe to allow some recovery time, and if recurrent, speaking with a therapist is suggested.

Be mindful and 'defuse' anxiety

Much suffering can arise from getting stuck in unhelpful ways of interacting with our thoughts or feelings. **Acceptance and Commitment Therapy** was introduced in Chapter 2. It outlines six key processes that can help us to develop more 'psychological flexibility', or our ability to adapt. We have talked about a few of them already, but we will continue to explore them here.

Dr Russ Harris, a medical practitioner and expert on Acceptance and Commitment Therapy, writes about the essence of this approach, namely: 'The greater our ability to be fully conscious, to be open to our experience, and to act on our values, the greater our quality of life because we can respond far more effectively to the problems and challenges life inevitably brings.'[3]

The six key processes are:

» **Defusion** and **acceptance**, which both help us open up to our thoughts and feelings.

» The **observing self** and **mindfulness**, which enable us to be more present.

» **Values** and **committed action**, which allow us to do what matters to us.[4]

These can be useful in taming stress anxiety, so let's look at each of them in more detail to help us work on our flexibility!

When we go to the gym we work on our flexibility. We also need to work on our psychological flexibility by opening up, being present, and doing what matters.

As mentioned earlier, mindfulness involves paying attention, in the moment, on purpose and in a non-judgmental way. An easy way to understand mindfulness is to watch a child playing. They are totally focused on what they are doing in that moment. When we are mindful, we become more relaxed, enjoy the moment, and are less likely to worry about the past or the future.

Mindfulness doesn't have to involve a great deal of time or effort. We can be mindful when doing everyday activities like eating and drinking. Using our senses is key, so that when eating a delicious piece of fruit, for example, we are more mindful of the colours, smell and taste. Or we might spend a few mindful minutes in nature, enjoying the trees or birdsong. We can even be mindful when doing household tasks!

There are also very effective mindfulness meditations, which incorporate being mindful of the sensations in different parts of the body (e.g. when sitting, noticing the sensations in our feet as they rest on the floor, and in our hands as they rest on our laps), being mindful of the breath (the feel of it, the movements of the chest) or being aware of the sounds around us.

When practising mindfulness, our thoughts often stray. This is very normal, as this is what the mind does. The aim is to bring our minds back to our senses and the meditation, and avoid getting tangled up in our thoughts or struggling with them. We can practise observing our thoughts or feelings without engaging with them, in meditation. This allows them to move through our mind, a bit like clouds floating across the sky.

Dealing with our wandering minds: When practising mindfulness, our thoughts often stray. This is very normal, as this is what the mind does! Simply observe them as they come and go.

And now onto the process of **defusion**. Fusion means being attached, and we can become 'fused' or very attached to our thoughts or feelings. Rumination or 'overthinking' is an example of this. Defusion is the opposite and means detaching from or stepping back from our thoughts and holding them gently rather than tightly. Defusion helps us realize that a thought is just a thought!

The following example from Russ Harris provides a powerful way to tame anxiety. Imagine your hands are your thoughts. If you cover your eyes with your hands for a moment and imagine what it would be like to go around all day like this, you'll realize that it would be very hard and you would miss out on a lot. This is like fusion. We become so caught up in our thoughts that we lose contact with the present moment, and we cannot function well. Now, rest your hands on your lap, which is like defusion. It feels more relaxed and you can engage in the moment and do what you need to do.[5]

Defusion is a way of managing troublesome thoughts. It involves noticing, stepping back, holding them less tightly.

There are many different strategies to defuse thoughts so that we don't get caught up with them. Russ Harris also suggests noticing a thought and saying, 'I am having a thought that ...' or imagining being near a stream, gathering up some leaves and twigs, and as you place each into the stream you also place a thought on it. The thought then floats off downstream.[6] Another strategy is to imagine a room with white walls and two doors. A thought comes in one door, and moves across the white wall, and then out the other door.

> **Use 'thought defusion' strategies:** Try saying 'I'm having a thought that ... Thanks, brain, for that thought!' Or sing the thought out loud!

As well as managing our thoughts through defusion, we also need ways to manage anxious feelings. The following strategy, called 'sitting with emotion', from Russ Harris, allows us to sit with anxious feelings and defuse them. If preferred, you can work through this with a therapist, or to practise the strategy, think about a recent time associated with mild (not severe) anxiety:

Get in touch with the situation and the feeling. Close your eyes and notice where the anxiety is felt in your body (e.g. in the chest or stomach). What shape or colour does it have? Does it have a temperature or texture? Then create some space or light around the feeling and sit with it for a while. Notice the breath, and breathe in and out. Imagine gently breathing into the feeling and keep breathing in and out to that spot in the body and see what happens with the feeling. When ready, open the eyes and come back to the room.[7]

Another process to look at is **acceptance**. Here this refers to making room for our thoughts and feelings, even uncomfortable ones like anxiety. It is often a challenge to accept our feelings, as we want to avoid feeling uncomfortable. The result is struggle and the anxiety may worsen. However, by staying with the discomfort and practising acceptance, the anxiety can lessen.

Acceptance and Commitment Therapy highlights two separate parts to the human mind: the 'thinking mind' and the 'observing mind'. You may know the thinking mind well with its constant stream of thoughts, but the observing mind may not be so familiar. The observing mind (or observing self) is the part of the mind that notices feelings and thoughts. Because of the observing self you can answer the questions, 'What am I thinking' or 'How am I feeling?'

This part of the mind allows us to 'step back' and observe things, but also remain separate from them. This part does not get hooked into what the thinking mind is saying. Understanding this concept and using the observing part of the mind helps us with defusion. We use it when we observe our thoughts and say, 'Thanks, brain, for those thoughts, but no thanks!'

The final two processes involve our **values** and our **actions**. Being aware of our values, or what we stand for, and living in accordance with them means that we invest our time and effort into what is important. Taking 'committed action' or 'doing what it takes', even if this brings up some discomfort, means recognizing that little change happens in life without action. Seeing a doctor or therapist, arriving at an appointment, reading self-help books, setting some goals or doing some regular meditation are all examples of committed action.

We need to take action, even when we don't feel like it: We do things we don't feel like doing all the time, such as cleaning. We don't actually have to feel like doing something to do it. And doing it can help us feel better!

A helpful way to think about anxiety is that it likes to jump into the driver's seat in our lives. Then we feel like a passenger getting thrown around in the back. All these processes and strategies help us to get back into the driver's seat in that moment. And so it is worth being familiar with them and putting them into practice.

Dealing with anxiety about illness

We all worry about illness at times, but when this worry impacts our daily functioning, then we need to consider whether it falls under illness anxiety disorder. This disorder understandably has become more prominent during COVID-19. It refers to being preoccupied with the fear of having, or the idea that one has, a serious disease. It is often based on a misinterpretation of bodily symptoms. For example, a regular pain might be interpreted as a serious illness, or a minor skin flaw might be misinterpreted as cancer.

Illness anxiety can trigger seeking reassurance from family, doctors or emergency department staff. There may be constant self-examination (checking over and over for breast lumps, for example) or self-diagnosis via internet searching. Or it may lead to avoiding having important regular check-ups due to fear of uncovering an illness.

Illness anxiety involves being fearful of serious illness. It can trigger checking or seeking reassurance.

Management of this anxiety involves seeing a doctor or therapist and learning more about it. A doctor can decide if any health checks are needed. The main behavioural therapies can assist with this disorder, in which the thinking trap of catastrophizing is often present, and thoughts often start with 'What if ...', for example, 'What if it is cancer?' These thoughts are future-based and are often related to a core belief of needing to feel in control or that 'bad things shouldn't happen'. The thoughts and the underlying beliefs actually heighten the anxiety.

We need to recognize the 'what if' thoughts and challenge them by saying 'What ifs aren't based on truth' or 'Where is the evidence?' Or we can observe the thoughts and recognize they are just thoughts: 'Thank you brain, but not today!' We can also work with the underlying beliefs. Sometimes we need to work on accepting that we can have some control, but not all of the time.

Doing an experiment to see what happens to the physical symptom when we keep checking (likely to increase) or noticing what happens to the level of anxiety symptoms when we keep searching the Internet can assist. The level will no doubt go up. Exposure is also used, and in this instance the exposure is not searching the Internet, not self-checking the body and making the gaps between medical appointments longer when they are for reassurance. Mindfully paying attention to what we notice with our senses, or being mindful whilst doing every day tasks can also assist.

How to quit rumination

Sometimes when we are anxious we can struggle with rumination (or repeating similar thoughts in our minds over and over), especially when exhausted or a mistake has been made. We can adopt some of the strategies outlined earlier in the chapter or consider:

» distraction with a walk, music or a movie

» asking whether the thoughts are true, or what thinking traps might be occurring (e.g. focusing on the negative or catastrophizing)

» using STOPP, both saying the word to interrupt the thoughts, or using stop in the following way: **S** for pause, **T** for take a breath, **O** for observe (what are the feelings and thoughts?), **P** for put it into perspective (is there another way of looking at it?) and another **P** for practising what works![8]

The 'Drop Anchor' technique, popularized by Russ Harris, helps anchor us in the moment and can disrupt ruminations and reduce worries. It works like this:

Acknowledge any thoughts and feelings, such as muscles feeling tight, worries or feeling overwhelmed. Then slowly push your feet into the floor, straighten your back and push your hands into your sides. Breathe slowly. You might think, 'Here's my body around my feelings.' And then loosen your body and wiggle your arms and legs, even dance around. Then engage with the world around you again, noticing what you can see, hear and touch.[9]

Antidotes to rumination: Include distraction, the word 'stop' and the 'Drop Anchor' technique.

Hypnotherapy and Narrative Therapy

Hypnotherapy involves helping the client achieve a deeply relaxed state (an altered state of consciousness). This is done through techniques to focus our attention and relax the body and mind. In this state, we are more open to suggestions or ideas. We can give suggestions about growing self-confidence and ways to manage anxiety.

Hypnotherapy sessions generally include learning self-hypnosis, a practical strategy that helps to reduce anxiety when used regularly. Specific suggestions to help manage general worrying, anxiety about performance (e.g. giving a talk) or panic episodes can be given, reinforcing many of the tools we have just talked about. In addition, phobias can be treated through exposure in the imagination via hypnosis.

Hypnosis can lead to deep relaxation and helpful suggestions can be given to assist with anxiety.

Make sure to seek out a qualified hypnotherapist. Hypnosis has been de-regulated in some countries, so look for therapists who are well trained to treat anxiety using a range of approaches and have solid training in hypnotherapy itself. The websites of professional hypnotherapy organizations can assist.

Narrative therapy provides another approach to assist with anxiety, as explored in Chapter 3 in relation to self-belief. In relation to anxiety, this approach involves:

» Externalizing the problem through our words, such as talking about anxiety as 'the anxiety is pushing me around'. We can visualize it as external to ourselves (e.g. as an animal or creature of some sort, in the middle of the floor).

» Being aware of the 'dominant' story related to anxiety, and constructing an 'alternative' story, for example of strength and resilience. We can ask ourselves how we have been pushed around by the anxiety, and how we have, even in a very small way, been able to stand up to the anxiety, and what qualities or skills this took.

Look for exceptions: There will always be exceptions to a dominant self-critical story. Just like panning for gold, we need to look for the flecks of gold, or the exceptions, amongst the dust.

5. Utilize self-help, and consider complementary therapies or medication

There are many good self-help resources available, including websites, books, podcast apps and online treatment and therapy programs. These often cover general information about stress and anxiety or may focus on a particular therapy. Make sure any of these that you choose are based on evidence and shown to be effective.

As mentioned, some complementary therapies or activities, such as yoga, massage or acupuncture, can be helpful. And supplements such as magnesium can also assist in anxiety. Personally, I find lavender tea calming, along with the process of making a pot of tea and sitting down in the garden to enjoy it! However, when anxiety is severe and getting in the way of what you need and want to do day-to-day, specific medications in combination with talking therapies may be suggested. Combining the two approaches can be more effective in severe anxiety rather than only using one, but medication should not be used without the talking therapies, as these create change for the long term.

We may feel fearful about using medication for anxiety. Having information can help a great deal. A range of medications may be used for anxiety (and depression), with the most common ones being selective serotonin reuptake inhibitors (SSRIs) or serotonin-noradrenaline/norepinephrine reuptake inhibitors (SNRIs). With any of these medications, it is very important to follow the instructions carefully. General guidelines include starting on a low dose to avoid side effects, building up the dose slowly, knowing that side effects often wear off after the first week or two, and that medications take time to take effect (from days to weeks).

Some of these medications can affect sexual functioning, so it is vital to discuss the best option with a doctor. And do not stop taking the medication suddenly; instead taper down the dose, always working with your doctor, as they can help monitor for any return of symptoms.

Let's summarize

Stress and anxiety are part of life, and so we are all familiar with them. At times they can significantly impact our wellbeing, and we have seen that during the pandemic. In this chapter we reviewed how the nervous system is involved in stress and anxiety and explored the various causes.

We delved into strategies from the various psychological approaches and identified a range of ways to deal with stress and anxiety, from reviewing lifestyle, reducing our stress bucket, to practising mindfulness. These are helpful for all of us in improving our mental health and wellbeing.

Talking with a trusted person or therapist means we are not taming anxiety alone. Identifying issues related to the stress and anxiety, and problem-solving some of them can help. Working on reframing unhelpful thoughts and on helpful actions can make a difference, whether via self-help resources or with a therapist. Practising self-compassion and using humour are essential.

We looked into anxiety disorders that may impact some of us and affect our day-to-day functioning, including illness anxiety disorder.

One particular approach may not suit everyone experiencing anxiety, so it is worth exploring a range of strategies to find out what fits you best. The brain is constantly changing, and practising different strategies helps to rewire the brain and create more flexibility, and ultimately helps us flourish.

Here are the keys from this chapter:

» Use breathing or meditation techniques.

» Grounding can be useful.

» Work with problem-solving.

» Allocate worry time each day, and put worry aside at other times.

» Avoid avoidance and use exposure.

» Use cognitive strategies to tame anxiety.

» Carry a 'taming panic' card.

» Deal with your wandering mind.

» Use 'thought defusion' strategies.

» Remember to take action, even when you don't feel like it.

» Antidotes to rumination include distraction, the word 'stop' and the 'Drop Anchor' technique.

» Look for exceptions to any dominant self-critical stories you have.

5

Adapting to change and challenge

"

Nothing endures but change.

— Heraclitus

Life is all about change! The various changes as we move through life can be exciting and wonderful. Thinking about getting a driver's licence or moving out of home, or our first main relationship or being married can trigger positive thoughts and feelings. However, managing change in life and various challenges that cross our path can also be stressful.

Looking at managing change and challenges is particularly relevant given the pandemic, which has created many changes in our lives, at home, at work, in our relationships and in our communities. It has also generated many challenges and, sadly, heartache, all of which have created a great deal of stress and anxiety.

Many of us have not seen anything like COVID-19 in our lifetimes.

At the centre of this period of change and challenge has been uncertainty about life and the future. During the pandemic many people have reported that they have felt empty, unmotivated or have experienced a sense of stagnation or numbness. Usual experiences that previously sparked joy no longer did so. Sociologist Corey Keyes coined the term 'languishing' to describe this experience. Languishing is not a single emotion, nor a mental illness, although having had anxiety or depression in the past might have made us more prone. Rather, it is a whole series of distressing feelings, and is the opposite of flourishing.[1]

In this chapter we will consider why change, challenge and uncertainty can be difficult to navigate. We have seen the exhaustion resulting from the pandemic, natural disasters and financial pressures in recent years. As a result, we will also consider the issue of burnout in this chapter.

Although humans don't particularly like change or uncertainty, we actually have the capacity to adapt well. The pandemic is a good example. We have seen people adapt to working from home, finding new work when jobs have been lost, home-schooling children or wearing personal protective equipment full-time in health care.

More than ever, understanding the impacts of change and various challenges on our mental health and wellbeing, having strategies to manage change and uncertainty, and strategies to maintain or improve our wellbeing are vital to flourishing.

About change and transition

Change is defined as an act or process through which something becomes different, while **transition** is the process or period of changing from one type to another.[2] Change and transition in life can be exciting and uplifting, but also very stressful at times, and involve an array of emotions including fear and grief. It can be especially hard to deal with the related uncertainty in life, as we all tend to like a sense of control and security.

During our lives, we experience change related to periods of life or transitions in our various roles. There are many transitions associated with the different life stages. Examples include moving in with a partner, getting a job, having children, divorce or retirement, to name a few. There can be change associated with gains in life such as a new house; situation or event-related transitions such as migration or job promotion; and illness-related transitions such as a diagnosis of chronic illness.

> Amali was 30 years old when she was diagnosed with an autoimmune condition. She had just started a new job in marketing, had met a new partner Beth, and was excited about moving into her own apartment, which she had just purchased. The diagnosis came at a time of transition in her life and involved more change. She had to see various specialists, have many investigations and begin treatment.
>
> Amali found that she wasn't sleeping well, was worried about keeping her job and relationship, and paying the mortgage and began questioning what her future might hold. She had dreams of travelling and having a family and feared these dreams might not happen. Her mother offered emotional and practical support and suggested that Amali see a therapist to talk more about all the challenges and how she was feeling.

We will come back to Amali a little later. Now, we are going to talk about the pandemic in more detail and then look at the strategies that might help us cope with change and transition.

The pandemic

The COVID-19 pandemic has been the most severe pandemic since the 'Spanish flu' in 1918. We first became aware of its presence in our communities in early 2020, and it continues to exert an impact on us in different ways.

Research on its effects on women's mental health and wellbeing is still scarce. One research paper concludes that the pandemic 'has affected women much more profoundly than men, both as frontline workers and at home. Financial crisis is ... developing and as a consequence mental health issues are likely to grow'.[3] We saw a rise in mental health issues and in domestic violence impacting women.

At the start of the pandemic, I asked my Facebook followers what they were most worried about. They spoke about:

» worry about family and friends getting sick, especially elderly parents, grandparents or children with health issues
» scarcity or lack of items at the supermarket
» loss of jobs or income and managing to pay the rent and other financial commitments
» dealing with conflicting information in the community
» concern surrounding the long-term repercussions and that life may not be the same
» worry about adolescent children who were isolated from friends and missing important milestones (school formals, gap years).

This question was asked at the start of the first lockdown in Australia, in March 2020, and although lockdowns were not mentioned as a specific stressor, they then became part of lives and created their own stress. With all the changes that have occurred since early 2020, many of us found ourselves feeling low in mood or worrying a great deal.

As explained in Chapter 4, when we feel a sense of threat to our safety or our regular life, or to the wellbeing of others, we can go into the fight, flight or freeze response. This is when our mind senses a threat and responds with adrenaline flowing through the body, causing all the physical and mental symptoms of stress and anxiety. When this response happens, we can experience a range of emotions or physical sensations, which can feel very uncomfortable, even overwhelming at times. These might include shock and disbelief (denial); stress, worry, anxiety and difficulty relaxing; feeling overwhelmed and a sense that the world is falling apart; or racing negative thoughts.

Physical signs of stress and anxiety, such as rapid heart rate, shallow breathing, sweating or nausea, along with tiredness, lethargy, fatigue and sleep difficulties might occur. We might also have difficulty concentrating, remembering or thinking logically; feel sad or tearful, irritable or angry; or feel disconnected from others and lonely.

Contributing to these experiences has been the shake-up of our day-to-day life, routines and standard social practices due to physical distancing, lockdowns and spending more time working from home. Many health care workers isolated themselves from family to protect them. And importantly, there may have been a challenge to what we value and our sense of identity and meaning in life throughout the pandemic.

The pandemic has involved change and uncertainty, and a threat to safety. A range of emotions and responses resulted.

When we face uncertainty, we instinctively try to control what is happening in our world. For example, we like routines, not only to get things done but to have a sense of certainty.[4] Routine can help, but as already mentioned, we cannot control everything. We certainly found this out during the pandemic!

In addition, we may have experienced a sense of loss during the pandemic, possibly due to separation from family in aged care facilities or interstate or overseas; cancelled weddings and celebrations; loss of job or independence; or loss of health. Loss means there is grief, and this has also played a significant part of the distress during the pandemic.

Despite all these challenges, the pandemic has led to some unexpected outcomes. Many of us reviewed our values and perhaps made decisions to spend more time with family, change working habits or simplify life. Many of these positive changes have continued.

Managing change and transition

Let's talk about how we can adapt to change and transition generally, and cope with some of the associated challenges. When there is a change, we tend to evaluate whether the change is relevant to our wellbeing and our goals, and how confident we feel in managing the situation.

Here are some points that can specifically assist you in adapting to change. The ideas are taken from some of the therapies we have already discussed:

» Focusing on what is important in life, and ensuring any goals are in line with your values. Maybe re-establishing some goals.

» Expressing your thoughts and feelings associated with the change, such as talking with family members, a colleague or a therapist. Or expressing your thoughts and feelings in your journal.

» Using personal strengths as a resource to assist with coping and adapting.

» Having structure and routine to the day and week, which can be reassuring.

» Ensuring pleasant and relaxing activities are scheduled into the week.

» Gathering support from others and connecting.

» Managing stress via lifestyle measures such as regular exercise, and fostering positive emotions such as gratitude, even for very small things in life.

» Focusing on what you can control or choose to act on and being more flexible in your thinking about what you can't control, and choosing to let these things go.

And some more!

» Problem-solving issues which arise as part of the change or transition, and sometimes using a 'wait and see' approach.

» Being aware of unhelpful thinking patterns such as black-and-white thinking or catastrophizing, which might impact levels of anxiety and mood, and working on more helpful or optimistic thinking.

» Being aware of underlying beliefs that might influence your thoughts and feelings during the period of change. These might include, 'I should always be in control' or 'Bad things should not happen to me'.

» Practising mindfulness to reduce stress and help you become less hooked by worries about the future.

» Finding meaning in the change and new roles; for example, recognizing what is important to you in life, or finding alternative work practices to have benefits.

» Fostering acceptance of change as it is part of life, and practising defusion techniques that assist with managing uncomfortable feelings.

» Regularly checking-in with yourself to see how you are doing, and practising self-compassion.

There are many keys to adapting to change: Managing stress, self-care, gathering supports, problem-solving issues and finding meaning in the change may assist.

Interpersonal Therapy offers some useful insights. This therapy is based on the idea that symptoms we might have are influenced by interpersonal issues. It identifies potential 'problem areas', including times of change in life, loss and grief and interpersonal conflicts, and helps us work through them.

Narrative Therapy can also assist with adaptation to change and role transition. The metaphor of a journey is often used to describe change and transition, and our personal strengths can be drawn upon to help navigate the journey. A technique called 'migration of identity' looks at the phases we go through in reincorporating our own identity into our lives after significant change, for example, migrating countries or divorce. Note that our journeys are rarely smooth, and there will be ups and downs, but the final phase is a period of readjustment.[5]

Hypnotherapy may also assist in coping with change or transition. Note, too, that we will look more at loss and grief in Chapter 6 and later explore specific issues associated with loss and grief, such as relationship breakdown (see Chapter 9) and coping with ageing or chronic illness (see Chapter 12.)

But let's come back to Amali for a few moments:

Amali saw a therapist and shared her thoughts and feelings. They discussed the changes in her life, physically, emotionally and practically, and the associated loss and grief. Amali learnt to manage some of the catastrophic thinking that had crept in, and to focus more on the moment rather than on 'what ifs'. She organized to do more work from home, shared her concerns with her partner, and engaged in more self-care activities.

Burnout

When I recently asked Facebook followers about how they were travelling in relation to the pandemic, the main response was 'exhaustion' from maintaining caring roles (children and elderly parents), and managing changes related to work, such as job loss and working from home. Hearing about this exhaustion, I started to question the current rates of 'burnout'.

It is reported that there is currently 'a global epidemic of burnout'. The World Health Organization describes burnout as involving feelings of exhaustion, increased mental distance from one's job, and decreased professional efficiency.[6] Burnout is also defined as a negative psychological syndrome that develops in response to chronic stressful work demands.[7]

Recent research has noted that burnout is not limited to formal work conditions and can occur in parents or carers. Women are at greater risk than men, and younger people are also more at risk.[8] Burnout is often diagnosed as depression, but it is not the same. It may also be confused with 'Myalgic Encephalomyelitis Chronic Fatigue Syndrome' due to the exhaustion, but this has its own range of symptoms.

The main symptoms reported by those experiencing burnout are exhaustion and cognitive problems. In addition, indifference or a lack of empathy, anxiety and depression symptoms, irritability and anger, sleep disturbance, lack of motivation or passion, impaired performance, withdrawing from social activities, physical symptoms, emotional lability and inability to feel (sense of depersonalisation) can also occur.[9] The work factors that may contribute include excessive hours, overly complex or relentless tasks, role issues, high levels of responsibility and uncertainty, lack of downtime at work, a perceived lack of control or support, and demands of technology and changing technology. An expectation of availability 24 hours a day via phone or email may contribute. The workplace environment can also contribute (such as noisy open offices or a toxic culture).[10]

It is thought that burnout is more likely when there is marked stress plus certain personality factors. Perfectionism has been identified as a risk factor. Treatment involves addressing all issues contributing to burnout, for example reducing various causes of stress, anxiety and managing perfectionism (see Chapter 6).

In burnout, our autonomic nervous systems are activated and hormones such as cortisol are released in the body to try to overcome the cause of stress. When this part of the nervous system remains activated for a long period, the growth of new nerve cells in the brain and neuroplasticity are limited.[11] Our immune system does not function as well so we may develop more infections, and inflammation can occur within the body.

There is a difference however, between burnout and 'burning out'. Many people are feeling chronically stressed and exhausted but are able to readily recover. When burnout occurs, recovery is also possible, but a significant reset in life may be needed.

Burning out and burnout are characterized by exhaustion, and are wake-up calls to reset in life.

Recovery includes managing stress related to work, including having appropriate training, supportive management and good conflict resolution procedures. Having meaningful work is important. For carers, reviewing self-care, gathering support (practical, professional), sharing the load and ensuring time-out are vital.

A team at the University of Sydney, including psychiatrist Dr Gordon Parker and PhD candidate Gabriella Tavella, have found that the first steps in recovery are to identify the burnout, then reflect on how it came about and the best ways to deal with it. They have identified six useful strategies for burnout:

1. talking to someone and seeking support (family, friends, doctor or therapist)
2. walking or other exercise
3. mindfulness and meditation
4. improving sleep
5. addressing perfectionism
6. changing your work situation based on individual needs and what is doable, recognizing there may be financial or other limitations (time off, reduced hours or changing work role).[12]

Ways to address burnout: Prevention is important, and adopting some or all of the six measures suggested above will assist.

Coping with natural disasters

At times we are affected by natural disasters, such as fires, earthquakes or floods. We may be familiar with 'disaster survival plans', but not so familiar with having a 'mental health survival plan'. It is important to be psychologically prepared.

At the time around the threat, we need to focus on the emergency advice given by the experts. We also need to be prepared that we may experience stress and anxiety and might need to calm our breathing as well as our thoughts. Thoughts that minimize or catastrophize the threat can occur, so it is helpful to focus on more realistic thoughts such as, 'We are going to follow our plan through step by step'.

We need a 'mental health survival plan' when facing natural disasters.

In other words, the three steps involved in being psychologically prepared are:

1. Anticipate that we will feel worried and anxious.
2. Identify the specific feelings and thoughts you are having.
3. Manage them with breathing and calm self-talk.[13]

As a disaster unfolds, humans tend to go into survival mode, doing what needs to be done. Once the threat has passed, we can stay in this mode for some time and experience a range of physical symptoms, behaviours, thoughts and emotions. Here are some examples:

» Being hyper-alert all the time, not sleeping and being tired or exhausted.

» Feeling numb, irritable, anxious, panicky or depressed.

» Feeling disorientated or confused.

» Possibly having strong recollections of the event or nightmares.

» Withdrawing from others or keeping very busy.

It is important to remember that these responses, even though they can be very distressing, are normal and can last for days or weeks. Here are some strategies to help with coping with an emotional response to disaster:

» Recognize that you have been through a very distressing experience and focus on feeling safe in the first instance.

» Avoid overusing alcohol or other drugs.

» Share your feelings, if you wish to, with support people.

» Let family and friends know about what you need practically and emotionally.

» Maintain a normal routine and do some things you enjoy.

» Resting when you can and use relaxation techniques.

» Eat well and do some exercise.

» Problem-solve what you need to be doing.

» Be aware that recent trauma may stir up memories from past traumas, and aim to keep these memories separate.

» Seek professional help if need be.[14]

Coping with natural disasters: There are many strategies to help us cope with a disaster. Review the list above and identify the most helpful ones. Write them down in your journal if helpful.

Disaster can involve grief following the loss of loved ones, property or animals. Many of the above strategies will be useful and more information on grief can be found in Chapter 6. Some individuals may have a severe or persistent reaction to related trauma. If significant distress lasts more than a few weeks, then please seek help from a doctor who can assess the situation. Following a disaster, some of us may go on to develop depression or post-traumatic stress disorder. Refer to Chapter 6 on depression and Chapter 10 on post-traumatic stress disorder.

Let's summarize

Life is full of change and transition, which can be exciting and challenging. It can involve gains as well as losses, and associated grief can add to distress. To manage change, we need to be patient and compassionate towards ourselves. Expressing the full array of feelings and drawing on their strengths can assist, as can coping skills.

The pandemic and recent natural disasters have been very challenging, especially due to the related life changes and uncertainty about the future. Humans are adaptable and a range of strategies have helped us to adapt, and can continue to do so. These include gathering all forms of support and problem-solving related issues. Allowing time and practising self-care are vital.

In terms of adapting to change, it is important to address any related loss and grief, and incorporate new aspects of our identity due to the changes. We also need to be mindful of burning out or burnout, with its signature exhaustion and impact on our functioning. The aim is to prevent or recover from it. Some of us will seek psychological support, and various approaches used can help us cope.

Having a mental health survival plan for natural disasters can help us be more psychologically prepared, and strategies such as focusing on safety, support and self-care are advised. At times mental health issues may complicate such trauma and professional assistance might be needed.

Remember, too, that change and transition can provide opportunities for self-awareness and growth. We saw this with the story of Amali. Equally, it can help to see the pandemic as 'an opportunity to build better, stronger, more resilient societies that could bring relief as well as hope'.[15]

Let's have a look at the keys from this chapter:

» There are many keys to adapting to change: managing stress, self-care, gathering supports, problem-solving issues and finding meaning in the change.

» Burnout prevention is important, and adopting some or all of the suggested six measures (p. 128) will help.

» Share your feelings about natural disasters if you wish to, practise self-care, maintain a regular routine, problem-solve what you need to and seek some professional help.

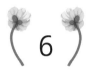

6

Overcoming depression and distressing emotions

"

Often we look so long at the closed door that we
do not see the one that has been opened for us.

— Helen Keller

This chapter will explore our mood or overall state of mind, and a range of distressing emotions. We will look at factors that affect mood, and in particular address depression. A number of keys to improving mood will be explored, and these keys can also be valuable for all women in fostering a greater sense of health and wellbeing.

We can all feel sad or low in mood at times, but we generally manage to get through the low times by using strategies that we know can help, such as talking to a friend or increasing our exercise. However, when our mood is persistently low over days and weeks, and significantly impacting our lives, we need to consider whether depression may have emerged. Depression is a common life experience and can occur at any age, especially at times of transition. A risk with depression is self-harm and suicidal thoughts, and it is important to manage these. Fortunately, depression is often fairly short-lived and uncomplicated, resolving in weeks or months, and there are many approaches and strategies that can assist.

Let's start by understanding mood generally, and depression in particular, and exploring strategies to improve these so that we can flourish. We will also explore grief and guilt in this chapter, and then loneliness, resentment and anger, and self-harm in the next chapter.

Many of the strategies highlighted in this chapter are helpful to our day-to-day wellbeing as well, so even if the 'negative' emotions aren't having a great deal of impact, the various keys can still be helpful to know about and can play a preventative role by improving mental wellbeing.

Understanding mood

Our mood is part of our overall sense of mental health and wellbeing, and our ability to flourish. Mood can be defined as 'a disposition to respond emotionally in a particular way that may last for hours, days, or even weeks, perhaps at a low level and without the person knowing what prompted the state'.[1] In other words, it is our predominant emotional state at a particular time. We often talk about being in a good, okay or bad mood, or being moody. This reflects that mood may be broader than one emotion.

Mood may echo particular emotions, especially happiness and sadness. Equally, fear or anxiety, which we addressed in the last chapter, as well as grief, resentment, anger or loneliness may impact mood. Mood itself can affect how we think, feel and behave, and can impact our motivation, social interactions, our memory and our perceptions.

Let's consider the various influences on whether we feel happy or sad in a particular moment. Our mood probably results from an interplay between a number of factors that are either external to us (such as employment situation) or internal (such as our personality). Our genetics, nutrition, level of exercise or sleep, presence of physical or chronic illnesses, various hormonal influences or drugs/medications may all influence mood. Psychological factors impacting mood include stress, our personality, thinking styles and impact of past experiences. Social factors include housing issues or poverty, relationship issues and level of social supports. Being isolated from others plays a role. Various cultural and spiritual or religious factors may also have an influence, as well as gender or sexuality concerns.

Being aware of these influences can enable us to consider whether they are playing a significant part in our lives or affecting our mood. A good place to start is to track your mood over a few weeks via a diary or a mood tracker app. Notice what your mood is, how strong it is (e.g. 0 for no sadness, and 10 for maximum sadness), and what is happening at the time. Keeping a diary like this can lead to surprising results, such as seeing that there are some better days and how often these are occurring, and that your mood may be worse when you're tired or stressed, for example. A good place to keep a record is in your journal.

Understanding your mood and what influences it are important. That way you can work on managing those influences, and achieve greater wellbeing as a result.

About sadness and depression

All of us experience sadness, often related to difficult life events. Feelings of sadness or brief depressive feelings are part of day-to-day life, but when a depressed mood persists and significantly impacts how we function, it may be related to depression. There are terms like 'clinical depression' or 'major depressive disorder' — we are going to simply say 'depression'. It is important to recognize depression so that it can be addressed.

Depression is not due to the same things in every woman. It can arise from a whole range of factors. We know life events can play a significant role in the development of depression, but we don't fully understand what is happening within the brain. There are various theories, but some of this research has been challenged in recent years, in particular our understanding about the chemical messengers or neurotransmitters in the brain and depression. What we do know is that the nervous system is complex with a multitude of connections between nerve cells and numerous cell processes involved, representing a whole ecosystem. Chemical messengers (including serotonin, noradrenaline, dopamine and gamma aminobutyric acid) play a part in brain functioning. Our reproductive hormones (see Chapter 8) and the stress hormones also influence the brain and its chemistry.

There is also a theory that depression somehow disrupts or damages some of the nerve connections, causing issues with memory and concentration. And interestingly, the role of inflammation in the body and mind in relation to depression is currently being researched, and we need to question whether aspects of our lifestyle (such as diet, lack of exercise, or chronic stress or trauma) may be contributing to this.

Risk factors include having a history of depression in the family, past depressive episodes, severe or chronic illness (e.g. heart disease or cancer), and loss and grief due to relationship breakdown or loss of a partner due to death. Trauma from childhood, sexual assault or intimate partner violence may also contribute to depression, along with issues related to gender or gender identity and sexual orientation. There may be difficulty in acceptance or social stigma, body dissatisfaction or bullying.

We are particularly vulnerable to sadness and depression at times of change in life, such as when changing jobs, moving house, relationship break-up or retirement. And women are also vulnerable at times of hormonal change, such as puberty, pregnancy, post-childbirth and menopause. We will look into hormonal influences in Chapter 8.

Depression is common, especially at times of transition in life. Women can be particularly vulnerable at times of hormonal transitions.

As mentioned earlier, we all have a negative bias, or a tendency to focus on negative thoughts (see p. 30). But negative thoughts can become a trap at times, with one negative thought generating more negative thoughts, and potentially triggering a downward spiral in mood. In addition, when there is depression, there is greater risk of anxiety, substance use (often to self-treat the symptoms) or problems such as gambling. Anxiety itself can also trigger depression.

No two women have the same story or experience when impacted by depression. Let's share a couple of stories about women experiencing depression:

Janie worked in a good job and was happily living with her partner, Josh. They were both thrilled when Janie became pregnant. She had always wanted to be a mother and the pregnancy went well. The delivery, however, didn't go as she hoped, and after the birth she started to feel 'blue'. These feelings did not go away, and after settling in at home Janie found herself feeling guilty as she thought that she should be 'over the moon' with happiness. The depression wouldn't shift and the anxiety was worsening too. A few months later Janie saw her doctor with the baby and started to cry.

Denise worked as a teacher her whole career, and when she and her partner Li both retired, Denise believed that 'their time' had finally arrived. They moved to the coast and settled into a new community, enjoying walking together, playing cards with friends, and some trips away. Then Li became unwell and was diagnosed with bowel cancer. Their lives were suddenly on a new path, and six months later Li died. Twelve months later Denise sought out a therapist, as her grief was still very intense and her mood extremely low.

Both Janie and Denise were experiencing depressed mood, very much related to their life stage and after very challenging events. Both recovered well, as we will find out later in the chapter.

Here is some information about general experiences with depression:

» Depression is one of a number of issues we can have with mood. Some mood problems are unique to women, such as premenstrual dysphoric disorder or depression around menopause (covered in Chapter 8). We can also experience dysthymia and bipolar disorder (covered later in this chapter).

» Women are diagnosed with depression almost twice as often as men. About 5 per cent of adult women will be diagnosed in any given year, and about one in seven women will be impacted over their lifetimes.[2,3]

» Although women mostly experience depression from their mid 20s, it can impact females of any age.

» About 10 per cent of women are diagnosed with depression while pregnant (referred to as perinatal depression) and up to 15 per cent of women are diagnosed with depression after the birth. This is more common in women who have experienced depression in the past or are being impacted by past trauma, substance use, social isolation, lack of support, challenging relationships or significant stress in life.[4]

» Perimenopause, or the time around menopause, is associated with increased risk of depression (see Chapter 8).

» Other conditions may co-exist with depression, such as anxiety, eating disorders, substance-related issues or borderline personality disorder (to be discussed shortly).

» Suicide is a significant risk with depression.

When diagnosing depression, the main features being looked for are ongoing low mood or loss of pleasure or interest in activities that were previously enjoyed. Further signs of depression might be struggling with eating or sleep (too much or too little), fatigue or low motivation, poor concentration or worse memory than usual, or feelings of hopelessness or guilt. We may also withdraw from relationships, have a lower libido than usual, be very self-critical, become over-involved with work or complain of feeling irritable. There may be self-harming behaviours or suicidal thoughts.

Symptoms of depression include persistent low mood or loss of interest or pleasure. Our thoughts and feelings, along with sleep, eating and energy may be affected.

There are tools available to aid diagnosis, such as the Patient Health Questionnaire (PHQ-9) or the Depression Anxiety and Stress Scale, and a doctor or psychologist can assist us in confirming whether a diagnosis can be made.

If concerned about depression: There are screening tests available online, but these can only indicate that depression 'may' be present. The next step is to speak with a doctor or mental health professional.

Other potential causes of disturbances in mood are dysthymia, adjustment disorder and bipolar disorder. **Dysthymia** refers to a persistent depressed mood for at least two years (including several related symptoms such as changes to sleep or appetites). **Adjustment disorder** can be triggered by a severe psychological stress (such as relationship breakdown). Emotional symptoms of distress may arise and interfere with functioning, but mostly they do not last more than six months. It may involve depression or anxiety symptoms.[5]

In **bipolar disorder** there are strong changes in mood and energy. There are periods of depression, and elevated mood or mania, often with agitation and overactivity, racing thoughts, little need for sleep and rapid speech. The changes in mood can last a week or more, and affect functioning, thoughts and behaviour. Bipolar disorder needs long-term management, which may include medication and psychological therapies. If you are concerned about symptoms that seem to fit with bipolar disorder, it is important to see a doctor for further assessment.

Depression may co-exist with a whole range of other mental health problems. Let's mention a few here:

» There can be lifelong mental health problems that affect interpersonal relationships, mood and behaviour in relation to

borderline personality disorder. There is often depression, and individuals also experience persisting struggles with relating to others and with a sense of self. There may be impulsive behaviours (such as self-harm or substance use) and difficulties regulating emotions, resulting in mood swings. Fear of abandonment in relationships is strong and can lead to self-harming or suicidal behaviours. There is often a history of trauma or issues with attachment to caregivers (see Chapters 7 and 9), or the origin may be genetic.[6]

» **Post-traumatic stress disorder** may follow exposure to a traumatic event. The trauma may involve injury, threatened death or sexual violence. It can result in a range of symptoms (see Chapter 10).

» **Complex post-traumatic disorder** is a relatively new term describing reactions that are typical of individuals exposed to chronic trauma (rather than acute trauma) from which escape is difficult (such as childhood sexual or physical abuse or intimate partner violence). The reactions are similar to post-traumatic stress disorder, but there are additional symptoms (see Chapter 10).

We will come back to these issues and their treatment in later chapters.

How to deal with low or depressed mood

All of us experience low mood at times, and some will experience persistent low mood due to depression. Many of the strategies highlighted in this chapter are helpful to know about to manage our mood and enhance wellbeing generally.

Maintaining a positive mood is a challenge because of our natural tendency towards negative thinking. Watching out for danger has helped us survive, and this is why we tend to look out for the negative in things. As a result we have many more negative than positive thoughts. For this and other reasons, learning how to manage negative thinking is valuable for all of us.

We are going to consider six steps that can assist with depressed mood:

1. Attend to physical health, lifestyle and self-care.
2. Identify what to focus on and set some goals.
3. Tap into talking therapies (to manage thoughts, feelings and actions).
4. Work with strengths, gratitude, meaning and purpose.
5. Consider self-help, complementary therapies or the role of medication.
6. Develop a relapse prevention plan.

1. Attend to physical health, lifestyle and self-care

When mood is significantly depressed, it is important to take action early. We may be able to adopt strategies we know have helped in the past, and at times we will need to seek out some assistance, and a good place to start is to talk to a trustworthy person, be it a partner, a family member or a friend, or speaking with a doctor or mental health professional.

Having a thorough assessment and physical check-up is vital. A good assessment can help differentiate between depression and other issues and it is important to make sure there are no underlying physical issues triggering low mood, such as low thyroid gland function, vitamin deficiencies or anaemia. A good health check-up is part of the assessment, and this will mostly likely involve having some blood tests.

It is vital to have a thorough assessment and physical check-up if our mood is significantly depressed.

The doctor will also work on a collaborative management plan. This involves identifying the main issues related to the depression, talking about treatment goals and a plan for how to work towards these goals. The plan might involve support and education, lifestyle changes, or potentially seeing a therapist or taking medication if appropriate, and linking in with other supports, including social supports. A good plan also includes what to do in a crisis and strategies for preventing relapse in the future.

The management plan includes taking a look at lifestyle and self-care, and seeing if anything related is contributing to the depression, for example, not eating well, little exercise or not having exposure to a reasonable (safe) amount of sunlight (which provides us with vitamin D that helps maintain mood). As mentioned earlier, appetite can be affected in depression. We may eat more or less food, or perhaps turn to 'comfort' foods. Our brain needs good nutrition to function, so focus on regularly eating healthy foods.

Exercise has been shown via research to have a positive effect on mood and it contributes to brain growth. So it is a very accessible and effective strategy. Start where possible and use small steps, and gradually build up the exercise with time. Consider an early morning walk, as the morning light stimulates mood-lifting neurotransmitters in the brain and aids sleep at night.

It is also important to schedule some pleasurable activities each day. Do some planning and map out one day at a time. Slot in some easy-to-achieve activities (e.g. talking with a friend, heading to the gym, having coffee, gardening or watching a movie), so that there are some pleasant activities included in your weekly schedule. We need to do the activities, even if we don't feel like them, because better feelings and more helpful thoughts will often follow.

Take action on depression: We need to take action even if we don't feel like it, because we will feel better as a result.

Anxiety often occurs with depression, so taking some time out to relax is important. This might be watching a film, listening to music or walking at the beach. Perhaps review the various relaxation techniques described in Chapter 4. Remember, too, that getting out into nature has been shown to be helpful in depression and for improving sleep, whether that is time in the countryside or at the local park.

Time in nature is healing: Take some time to get out into nature, whether in a garden, walking in a park or at the beach. The sunshine, exercise and being mindful in nature can all assist recovery.

It is important to reduce the use of alcohol, cigarettes and other drugs when feeling depressed. They can worsen the depression and complicate life. And don't forget to regularly disconnect from phones, tablets or laptops. Our brain needs time away from being stimulated by technology, and it needs some silence too, such as we find in nature.

Trouble going to sleep, or waking up in the middle of the night or too early in the morning are often problems when our mood is depressed. **Improving sleep** aids recovery. Strategies that can assist include:

- » going to sleep at a regular time each night and avoiding sleep during the day
- » using regular ways to wind down before sleep (such as a warm shower or listening to calming music)
- » dimming lighting during this time (including brightness on screens), which is important for letting the brain know it is time for sleep
- » getting off screens at least an hour or two before bed
- » meditations to aid sleep
- » exercising during the day to ensure physical tiredness
- » avoiding too much caffeine during the day/evening, and alcohol at night
- » avoiding large, heavy meals in the evening
- » eating food such as bananas or warm milk, which can have a calming effect at night (because of the type of proteins in them).

2. Identify what to focus on and set some goals

Part of overcoming low or depressed mood is working on some of the issues contributing to the depression, whether internal (our ways of thinking and behaving) or external (interpersonal or work issues, finances, housing). We all share core needs of safety, satisfaction and connection. Depression may be triggered or worsened when these needs are not being met, such as basic housing and financial needs, some sense of contentment in life, or connection with others. There might also be internal factors such as our personality traits that contribute to depression, or our thoughts might tend to be more pessimistic than optimistic about life and ourselves. Continued pessimistic thinking is a risk factor for depression returning and so it is very important to address this.

A therapist will listen to our story and help us make sense of what is going on. They may suggest that you work on some short-term goals to begin with, such as improving sleep or doing some walking. Sometimes the tiredness that comes with depression can be a barrier to this or we might take on the idea that we need to feel like doing something to actually do it. As mentioned earlier, the important thing is to do the activity, even if you don't feel like doing it! When we have taken some action, we tend to feel better in ourselves.

Remember that sometimes we can take two steps forward and one back, and that is okay! It helps to start with very easy-to-do activities, breaking them down into small steps, and to include some activities that give us pleasure, such as phoning a friend. The planning would include working out when we feel most able to do this, having a prompt such as setting a phone reminder, and planning to speak for just a short period of time to begin with. And don't forget the celebration when the call is done!

Consider setting some short-term goals: Start with easy-to-do or pleasurable activities and take very small steps. Remember that sometimes we take two steps forward and one back, but we get there in the end!

3. Tap into talking therapies

In depression, our thinking can become more negative and trigger a downward spiral, worsening the feelings of depression. Thoughts may be self-blaming or self-critical. We might have thoughts such as 'It's all my fault' or 'I'm not good enough', or we may have a negative view of the world or our future.

These thoughts create a lot of distress, so having ways to deal with them is vital. We are going to look at different approaches to dealing with negative thoughts, and remember that these are not only helpful in depression but in dealing with our 'negative bias' in general, and improving mental wellbeing.

Again, **Cognitive Behaviour Therapy** can assist us in dealing with negative thoughts. This therapy was described in detail in Chapter 4, but here we are going to apply this approach to depression. At the essence of this therapy are the interactions between how we feel, think and behave. They all influence each other. The reality is that we all experience negative thoughts.

We all experience negative thoughts, especially when our mood is low or depressed. Learning skills to manage these thoughts is incredibly useful.

This approach involves becoming more aware of our thoughts by reflecting on them or writing them down in a thought diary or the journal. This is the first step. We then need to understand that some thoughts are helpful, and some positively unhelpful and untrue! This is because we all experience traps in our thinking (see p. 101). Common thinking traps in depression are black-and-white thinking (thoughts are one extreme or the other), labelling ('I'm a failure') or catastrophizing ('It's a disaster'). Once we learn to identify these traps and challenge unhelpful thoughts, we can then develop some more helpful ones. This then assists us to improve our mood!

Here is an example. We might think, 'I'll never be able to do this job, I'm hopeless at it'. The thinking traps of black-and-white thinking and labelling are evident here. Useful challenges include asking yourself, 'Am I being black and white, or too self-critical? Is this thought true, or is there another way to think about it? If a friend was saying this to me, what would I say to them?' In response we might come up with a more helpful thought such as, 'I am doing okay, learning a new job takes time'. This is also called **reframing**. The new thoughts don't have to be overly happy, simply more balanced or helpful.

Reframing is a vital skill: Notice negative thoughts and any thinking traps. Then do a 'reframe' or find a more helpful way to think about the situation.

Cognitive Therapy and mindfulness have been combined into **Mindfulness-based Cognitive Therapy**. Rather than challenging thoughts, this approach involves becoming more aware or mindful of our thoughts and feelings, and helps us relate to them differently.[7] It is important to recognize that our thoughts and feelings are part of our experience and give us lots of information, but that we are often 'totalized' by them. We are not our thoughts!

The aim is to get less caught-up or hooked on our thoughts, by viewing them as mental events that we can observe. A useful metaphor is to see our thinking as like the weather. A weather change comes in and then it passes. Our thoughts do the same.

Mindfulness-based Cognitive Therapy also encourages self-compassion, which involves using mindfulness to acknowledge our feelings rather than suppressing or avoiding them, and remembering that we are human and make mistakes. We also work on putting things into perspective rather than buying in to comparisons, and treat ourselves with the kindness we would give others feeling the same way.

Ideas from **Acceptance and Commitment Therapy** are also very useful when feeling depressed, as this approach takes up the idea of relating differently to our thoughts and feelings. As mentioned earlier, this approach suggests that we can become hooked on or 'fused' with negative thoughts, especially about the past. This can cause unpleasant feelings, which we might then try to avoid. Also, rumination or overthinking can occur. To reduce overthinking, we need to work on being less 'hooked' by our thoughts and feelings, and we need to not avoid uncomfortable feelings and ruminate less by focusing on the here and now (see p. 111).

Be less 'hooked' on thoughts: We are not our thoughts! When we research a topic via Google, one search might come up with hundreds of results. We don't pay attention to all of them, but choose the ones that look most helpful. We can do the same with our thoughts.

Narrative Therapy can also assist with mood. As explained in Chapters 3 and 4, the essence of this approach is that we create meaning in our lives with stories, made up of events over time. Some stories are more dominant than others and full of problems (e.g. 'I am a failure'). We sometimes forget that there are alternate stories, such as having a range of strengths or being competent at various things in life.

In addition, the person and problem tend to be seen as one and the same. For example, if we are being pushed around by depression we may view ourselves as being depressed, somehow weak, a nuisance or to blame, rather than a competent individual who is being affected by the depression. This can result in feeling helpless about taking action. We need to remember that we are human, travelling through life with all its challenges, and that change is always possible!

We create meaning in life with stories, some of them about ourselves, and some negative or self-critical. There are always alternative stories, full of strength and hope.

Narrative therapy invites us to consider a number of questions about depression, namely:

» How has depression impacted your view of yourself?

» Think of a time when in some small way you have been able to stand up to the depression and have stopped it pushing you around.

» What qualities, skills or abilities did it take for you to resist depression in this way?

» How can you use these qualities, skills, abilities or strategies in future to continue to challenge the depression?

» Think back through your life to other times when you were able to outsmart depression and describe what happened.

» What kind of person are you in the process of becoming, and what would your partner or a good friend say about this?[8]

These questions help us relate to the depression in a different way. We can then recognize that we are much more than the depression, and that we have many strengths and strategies to overcome it.

In this section, we have looked at a few different approaches to managing thoughts, behaviour and feelings. We are all individuals, so make a note in your journal about the approaches that seem to fit you best.

Perfectionism and procrastination

Let's bring some of these ideas together with the example of **perfectionism**, which involves wanting to do things extremely well or expecting the same of others. Rates seem to be increasing worldwide, so it is pushing many of us around. It can be a 'friend' at times by helping us do a good job, and a 'foe' at others by creating pressure.

Perfectionism may appear in different areas of our lives, including appearance, weight, fitness, how we perform at work or socially, cleanliness, music or sport. It can be involved in disappointment and depression in life, because it results in putting pressure on ourselves to meet really high standards. Perfectionism can drive high expectations, and a sense of not doing well enough, or not being enough, if not meeting those expectations.

The underlying beliefs involved in perfectionism can include needing approval from others, to be 100 per cent competent in life, and needing to feel in control. These beliefs lead to traps in our thinking, especially black-and-white thinking or catastrophizing: 'I must do things perfectly, otherwise I have failed' or 'It will be the end of the world if this doesn't go how I want it to'. These patterns also lead to self-critical thinking and defining our worth by how well we perform.

Perfectionism can lead to monitoring (checking appearance or cleanliness excessively), avoidance (such as avoiding decisions or social situations), and procrastination, hoarding or seeking reassurance. It can be a factor in anxiety or depression. It is a common trigger to peri- or postnatal issues (around or after the birth of a child), with a sense of wanting to be the perfect mother and finding this is really hard to measure up to as babies do things in their own way and time!

Perfectionism involves wanting to do things really well, making it hard to measure up to unrealistic standards. It is really an illusion!

So what can we do to make sure perfectionism works for us, rather than against us?

» Be aware of your own and others' expectations and check if they are realistic.

» Remember that doing things perfectly does not necessarily make others see us as more worthy.

» Take time to reflect and weigh up the pros and cons of being a perfectionist.

» Stop comparing yourself with others!

» Think about putting some time limits on different tasks, and work to the set time rather than doing the job perfectly.

» Notice unhelpful thoughts such as 'What would happen if I made a mistake occasionally; what is the worst thing that could happen?' Then challenge them and keep things in perspective.

» Be aware of any fears that are hiding behind perfectionism (fear of failure or of criticism), and work on the fears.

» Remember that very few things in life are perfect. Sometimes we need to aim for a 'middle path' in what we do, rather than an extreme.

» Dare to be average or do a 'good enough' job some of the time!

» Practise mindfulness, be kind to yourself and aim for flexibility.

Challenge perfectionism: Reflect on what might be driving it, and notice related thoughts and underlying beliefs. Challenge these, and experiment with doing a 'good enough' rather than a perfect job.

Take some time to write down any reflections in the journal or some of the tips that seem most helpful. Sometimes doing an experiment with behaviours can be useful too. For example, if we find ourselves always responding to text messages within a few minutes, experiment with not responding so quickly. We might predict that some people may notice the change, but it is likely that everyone will adjust!

Tied in with perfectionism is **procrastination**. This might be used to avoid a stressful situation, such as delaying a work project. Sometimes using distractions, like the internet or smoking, is a form of procrastination. Procrastination can also be related to high expectations, or it may stem from a fear of failure or criticism, self-doubt, a fear of uncertainty, a desire to be approved of by certain people in our lives or a desire to be in control of things.

It is important to reflect on what might be driving your procrastination and notice related thoughts and underlying beliefs, and work on challenging these. It can help to replace the word 'should' with 'choose', and if distraction is being used to avoid a task, consider whether the distraction comes at a cost.

We might need to set more realistic goals for ourselves, and plan to do tasks when we have more energy and motivation, such as first thing in the morning. Sometimes we also need to learn to sit with unpleasant feelings rather than using distraction (see the 'Sitting with emotion' exercise on p. 108).

4. Work with strengths, gratitude, meaning and purpose

Overcoming depression involves using our strengths. Refer back to Chapter 2 and the section on strengths, and consider which strengths might assist. The strength of perseverance, for example, can assist when dealing with a low mood, as we have to keep taking actions we know will help over time. Consider other strengths that might help in dealing with feeling depressed.

As mentioned earlier, our minds tend to focus on negative thoughts, so we have to work hard at fostering positive thoughts to experience good moods. Apparently, we need a ratio of three positive thoughts or experiences to each negative one to have a better mood. When depression is around, it can help to plan or create more positive experiences (e.g. seeing a friend, going for a walk), and tapping into happy memories or watching a comedy can also shift our thinking.

Another way to encourage more positive thoughts and feelings is by practising gratitude. Even when life is very challenging and we are feeling low, it is still possible to be grateful for things in our lives and this can help us to cope. As mentioned in Chapter 2, research suggests that to improve mood, we need to write down or say out loud three things that we are grateful for once a week.

Regularly tap into gratitude: Write down in your journal three things you are grateful for today. They can be small or large things (e.g. spending time in the sunshine, some kind words, or patting the dog).

Meaning and purpose in life are vital, and are often based on what we value (e.g. helping others or creating). Activities are part of life and meaning, and bring enjoyment and challenge, whether work, home or leisure-based. When mood, energy and motivation are low, meaningful pursuits are often dropped. However, it is important to keep them going or pick them up again, step by step. Refer back to Chapter 2 on meaning and purpose, and any reflections made in the journal.

5. Consider self-help, complementary therapies or the role of medication

As outlined in Chapter 4, there are many good self-help resources available, including online therapy programs (often based on Cognitive-Behaviour Therapy). Make sure they are based on evidence and shown to be effective.

We may also look to complementary therapies. Examples include various herbal medicines or supplements (generally used for milder depression). Due to side effects and interactions with other medicines, always discuss complementary medicines with a health practitioner.

There is evidence that fish oils (omega-3 supplements), vitamin B9 (folate) and vitamin B12 can have a beneficial effect on mood. Note that the fish oils are not to be used in bipolar disorder, or if taking blood thinner medications. Light therapy may assist with seasonal depression (also known as seasonal affective disorder, or SAD).

When depression is more severe, medications may be suggested alongside talking therapies. Combining the two approaches can be more effective than one alone. It is important to discuss any potential role of medications with your doctor. (Please refer back to p. 115 to read more about SSRIs and SNRIs.)

Very rarely we can feel more depressed in the weeks after starting medication, and if this happens, talking with your doctor is vital. Medication for a first episode of depression is generally continued for six to twelve months, but if there are repeated episodes, medication may be needed for a longer period.

6. Develop a relapse prevention plan

Depression can sometimes relapse or return. Many women will recover from depression and not experience another episode, but some will have a second episode and a smaller number will have a more chronic course. This is why it is important to have a relapse prevention plan in place to provide a few reminders about what to do if symptoms re-occur. There are three steps in developing a plan for managing depression relapse:

1. Identifying the early warning symptoms, such as difficulty sleeping, ruminating and withdrawing from friends.

2. Identifying possible high-risk situations for relapse, such as stress or being overtired, and considering coping strategies such as taking some time out or exercising.

3. Preparing an emergency plan, such as keeping an eye on thinking, getting support, making an earlier (or urgent) appointment with a doctor or using medication if that was helpful last time.

Notes related to these three steps can be made in your journal so you have a plan to refer to when needed.

Guilt and shame

The emotions of guilt and shame were introduced in Chapter 2. They are distressing, and may contribute to sadness or depressed mood, and complicate grief. Let's consider the following definitions from Brené Brown:

» **Shame** involves a focus on self, with thoughts like, 'I am bad' or 'I am a mistake', meaning that there is something 'inherently wrong with who I am'.

» **Guilt** relates to behaviours or actions, with related thoughts such as, 'I did something bad' or 'I made a mistake'.[9]

Guilt and shame are different. Guilt relates to actions and thinking, 'I did something wrong'. Shame involves a focus on self, with thoughts like, 'I am bad'.

Guilt can contribute to low mood. Earlier in the chapter we heard the stories of Janie and Denise. Guilt was playing a role in Janie's low mood and anxiety: 'I should be over the moon with happiness, and I'm not.' Denise felt guilty that she was alive when her husband had died, and that sometimes she didn't feel grief. These thoughts are not based on truth, and working with them relieved much of the distress.

Shame in particular can be related to depression, trauma and addictions. Sometimes women who have experienced abuse feel shame, but the abuse was not their fault. Responsibility lies with the perpetrator, and shifting blame to where it belongs is the first part of recovery. We will look at some of these issues in Chapters 9 and 10.

Guilt and shame can result in feeling disconnected or insecure, being self-critical, or setting unrealistic expectations. This is related to the underlying human need for love and belonging, to know we matter and that we are part of something. We try to fit in to what society tells us to do and it is extremely painful when we don't think we measure up or are not worthy.

There are some potential strategies for dealing with guilt and shame, including being mindful of the feelings and naming them, working through them rather than avoiding them, working with related thoughts and beliefs and practising self-compassion. If the thoughts are self-critical, then we can reframe them. Sometimes we do need to take responsibility for any mistakes, correct them and then focus on self-forgiveness. Connecting with others who can provide support may also assist.

> **Working through guilt and shame takes courage:** It might be helpful to write about your feelings in your journal or talk about them with a therapist. We are constantly learning in life, and dealing with the guilt or shame may be part of your learning and resultant change.

Grief

As we move through life, we experience various losses and grief, and this can feel very distressing.

- » **Loss** involves separation from something or someone that has meaning to us and to which we feel connected. This may be associated with death of a loved one or pet, or other losses such as a job or relationship.
- » Some losses are anticipated (such as losing a relative with terminal cancer), and some are disenfranchised, that is, not well acknowledged in society (such as losing someone who suicides).
- » **Grief** is the response to loss, and affects many aspects of us (physical, psychological, social, spiritual).

We may experience grief in a number of ways, via feelings, physical sensations, thoughts and behaviours. Feelings occur in no particular order, and it can feel like being on a rollercoaster. The emotions may include shock, numbness, sadness, anger, guilt, anxiety, loneliness, helplessness, yearning, despair, depression or relief (for the deceased in the ending of suffering). We may have a sense of disbelief or confusion, a sense of hopelessness or unreality.

Physical reactions include tiredness, breathing difficulties or muscle weakness. Behaviours can include crying and being restless. We may withdraw from family and friends, or have problems sleeping or eating.

The experience of loss and grief varies between individuals, and we may experience a whole rollercoaster of emotions.

Processing loss and grief takes time, sometimes a very long time. This may be because we have a strong attachment to the lost person. Therapist Dana Lerner writes that losing her child felt as though part of her was missing and that there was a hole in her heart. She started writing as a way of dealing with the pain, and while researching grief found a piece by psychiatrist Sigmund Freud, who also lost a child. He said that, 'the pain is always there, the way it should be. It's the only way to perpetuate a love we don't want to give up'. Dana realized that the attachment would never be lost and that the love would live on.[10]

Some experts talk about there being 'tasks' or work in grieving, including accepting the reality of the loss, working through the pain of grief, adjusting to an environment without the lost person or item (such as a house) and rebuilding your own life and identity. Loss and grief may also challenge our beliefs about the world and we need to process these, too.

In the past we talked about 'closure' or 'moving on', but we now know that it is vital to create continuing bonds or connections with the person or item that has been lost. To do this we focus on the meaning of the connection. For example, if we lose a parent, we might continue to contemplate what they would say or do in a particular situation to help guide us.[11] An extension of this idea is reconstructing meaning. An example might be doing something to honour the person, such as a memorial or fundraising for a cause.

General strategies for dealing with grief

It is important to pause a while to work through your emotions. During this process it is vital that you maintain self-care, including eating regularly and keeping to routines as much as possible. Avoiding alcohol or other substances is advised.

Grounding exercises can assist when feeling disoriented (see p. 93), as can simple things that you normally enjoy, such as taking a walk in nature, listening to a podcast or looking at a magazine. Reflecting on and using your strengths and resources to manage the loss and grief can assist. You might want to connect with others or have quiet time.

The concept of 'grief time' can be helpful, particularly once the acute grief has settled a little. This means allowing some grieving time each day, such as half an hour or an hour, to focus on the grief and have a cry, look at photos, or write in your journal. Outside this time it is okay to have less focus on the grief.

It can also help to create a folder or box about the loss and grief, with mementos and pictures that can be looked at whenever you choose. Considering how to manage celebrations or anniversaries is important. Whether you want to be alone or with others, it is important to be kind to yourself, choosing what you want to do and reducing expectations on yourself at those times.

Dealing with loss and grief: This involves looking after yourself and allowing some grief and non-grief time. You might need to rebuild your life and it can help to maintain connection with what has been lost in some way.

Author and clinical psychologist Julie Smith refers to the 'pillars of strength' that we need to work on to stabilize and rebuild our lives as we grieve. These are based on the work of the work of grief psychotherapist Julia Samuel, who speaks about the importance of:

» our relationship with the person who has died or finding new ways to feel close to the loved one, such as visiting the grave

» our relationship with self or self-awareness, using our coping skills and gaining support

» expressing grief

» time, and at the start taking it one hour or one day at a time

» mind and body self-care

» listening to our own needs and possibly setting limits or boundaries in relation to work or with others

» structure or routine

» focusing on our feelings and internal world.[12]

We all grieve in different ways, so drop any comparisons with others, and remember, there is no timeline for grief. If loss and grief are very distressing or your emotions are not easing over time, seeing a therapist may be helpful. Sometimes grief can be complicated because it remains intense over time, especially when the loss involves uncertainty or trauma. Occasionally depression can result or there may be issues related to the trauma. In these instances, seeing a doctor and a therapist is vital. They will listen and provide empathy, support and information.

Therapists use various grief counselling approaches. Grief is challenging because many losses are beyond our control, and because attachments are lost. There may be related losses, such as loss of financial security or a shared future. A therapist can guide you through these issues and also monitor how you are progressing, including checking for any risk of self-harm (as we are more vulnerable when grieving).

A therapist will also encourage reconnection with other people and ways to rebuild your identity. One tool from Narrative Therapy is particularly helpful in maintaining connection with a lost loved one. It encourages you to say 'hello again' to the person you are grieving, and means you can have an ongoing connection with them while still learning to live a life without them being physically present.[13]

To do this, ask yourself questions such as these:

» If you were seeing yourself through [deceased's name] eyes now, what would you notice about yourself that you could appreciate?

» What difference would it make to how you feel if you were appreciating this in yourself right now?

» What would they have said or done in certain situations?

If this section seems relevant, write down any reflections or useful keys in your journal.

Some final reflections

We are almost at the end of this chapter, and it is time to follow up Janie and Denise.

Janie and her doctor talked about her main concerns and together they shed more light on them. A physical check-up showed that Janie was low in iron after the birth, and this was addressed. They looked at the current routines with the baby, and ways to manage sleep, with Janie giving herself permission to rest during the day. They talked about the whole range of normal in relation to dealing with a young baby, and about dropping some of the high expectations. Janie was referred to a therapist for extra support and to work through a range of psychological strategies.

Denise sought grief counselling and was relieved to be able to share her thoughts and feelings. She was tearful in the first couple of sessions. The therapist explained the nature of grief and the whole range of emotions that might be experienced. This was reassuring. They talked about some practical ideas such as focusing on self-care, allowing grief time (and non-grief time) each day and connecting regularly with others. Together they explored some of Denise's thoughts related to the guilt and these were challenged. Denise was encouraged to reflect on how to form continuing bonds with her late partner, and she continued to meet with the therapist regularly for about six months. Her mood continued to improve over this time.

We are also going to reflect on **hope** at the end of this chapter. Hope is not blind optimism or wishful thinking, but rather a positive state of mind based on the expectation that positive outcomes will occur in our lives. It is also the action of expecting that our individual goals will come to fruition. It is a way of thinking and a behaviour that requires us to have the ability to apply a positive influence in our lives in order to achieve our goals.[14]

Having expectations that positive outcomes will occur, and taking action towards these, gives us hope.

It is important for us to feel a sense of hope because life is difficult and presents many challenges. By having a strong sense of hope we become more resilient and better able to adapt to change, as well as tackle our goals with a greater sense of optimism and enthusiasm. Hope is vital as it can generate creative thinking, courage and determination to overcome all sorts of challenges in life. Hopeful people are thought to experience better general health, increased determination, a greater sense of achievement and lower rates of depression.[15]

In fact, there is a particular form of therapy called Hope Therapy, which involves identifying and working towards goals, and sustaining the motivation to reach them through believing we can change. Part of the difficulty can be feeling too overwhelmed to start. Again, taking one small step at a time can help. Momentum and a sense of satisfaction then builds, helping us move to the next step. Hope Therapy also encourages people to be flexible in their thinking and approach (e.g. if one way doesn't work, then try a different way!).[16]

To foster hope: We need to take action (have the will) and believe we can instigate change (find a way).[17]

 Let's summarize

We have covered a lot of ground in this chapter and focused on understanding and managing depression, as well as guilt and shame, and loss and grief. We have considered depressed mood in detail, as it is a common and potentially serious problem.

Understanding depression and taking up some of the strategies we have covered can assist in overcoming it. Never underestimate the power of addressing lifestyle and self-care. Remember, too, that you are the expert on yourself and have many internal strengths and resources you can draw upon. Engaging in activities that bring a sense of meaning and purpose can assist your mood, too.

Working on managing your thoughts, feelings and behaviours is vital, and you can do this in many ways. We have looked at various strategies from a range of psychological approaches. One size doesn't fit all, so please choose the approaches and related strategies that seem to fit you best.

Seeking early input from a doctor and therapist may be helpful or necessary in dealing with depression. Working on your thinking is vital, as negative thinking worsens in depression and can hook us in. This does take work, but is well worth it, both to recover from depression, to prevent relapse and to flourish.

Hopefully some of the ideas in this chapter will help in dealing with depression or distressing emotions. Many of them will also help us to achieve a greater sense of wellbeing, especially during times of challenge or distress.

Feeling a sense of hope is so important, and if we work in small steps while maintaining compassion for ourselves, we can move forwards. As Victor Hugo said, 'even the darkest night will end and the sun will rise'. The keys provide a reminder of this hope.

- » If concerned about depression, there are screening tests available online, but these can only indicate that depression 'may' be present. The next step is to speak with a doctor or mental health professional.
- » Take action even if you don't feel like it.
- » Time in nature is healing.
- » Consider setting some short-term goals.
- » Reframing is a vital skill.
- » Be less 'hooked' on thoughts.
- » Challenge perfectionism.
- » Regularly tap into gratitude.

» Working through guilt and shame takes time and courage.

» Dealing with loss and grief involves looking after ourselves and allowing some grief and non-grief time.

» To foster hope we need to take action (have the will) and believe we can instigate change (find a way).

7

Dealing with other emotions and self-harm

"

The doors to the world of the wild Self are few but precious.
If you have a deep scar, that is a door. If you love the sky and
the water so much you almost cannot bear it, that is a door.
If you yearn for a deeper life, a full life ... that is a door.

— Clarise Pinkola Estes

In the last chapter we looked at a range of potentially distressing emotions and we spent time understanding the nature of depression, and approaches that may assist. We are going to consider some other emotions in this chapter, including resentment and anger. Two important strategies to manage these will be outlined, namely setting boundaries and being assertive.

We are going to explore loneliness and rejection, as these both have significant effects on our mental health and wellbeing. We will also learn about an additional approach called Dialectical Behaviour Therapy that can help us soothe ourselves at times of distress.

Importantly, this chapter has a focus on ways to prevent and manage suicidal behaviours and non-suicidal self-harm (behaviours deliberately hurting the body, such as cutting). It is written both for women in distress, and for anyone who is trying to assist. It offers information and some strategies to assist, but these do not replace emergency support or professional assistance. *So, if struggling with self-harm or suicidal thoughts, don't wait! Please seek help straight away.*

Let's start with looking at resentment and anger.

Resentment

Unfortunately, it seems that resentment is an emotion many women can relate to. Interestingly, resentment is related to envy, due to perceived unfairness or injustice. It is all about needs not being met and feels similar to frustration and anger.[1] The injustice may be true or imagined, and can relate to interactions with others or an experience.

Here is an example:

Josie picks up two of her children from out-of-hours school care, grabs a chicken for dinner at the supermarket and heads home. She finds her teenage child at home with her partner, who works from home. There are dishes on and in the sink, and the laundry is still full of sports clothing from the weekend. She pulls out all the school notices to deal with while preparing dinner, and feels her resentment rise up again. She takes the kitchen tidy bag out to the bin and swears as she throws it in.

Does this sound familiar? Common causes of resentment include constantly doing a lot of the work in a relationship or family, whether it is emotional work or practical jobs such as housework or child care, being the breadwinner or doing all of these at the same time! There may be challenges in the relationship such as communication issues (unhelpful ways of managing conflict such as blaming or hurtful words or behaviours), a power imbalance, leading to feeling unheard, overpowered or abused. A betrayal or infidelity (see Chapter 9), or becoming a carer in a relationship can trigger resentment.

When feeling resentful, we may be too angry or ashamed to talk about it, which allows the resentment to grow and it is then often expressed as anger. Resentment may lead to ruminations about the interaction or event, feelings of regret, avoidance of speaking up due to not wanting conflict or tense relationships. It can trigger feeling 'less than' or not enough.

Resentment relates to a sense of unfairness and injustice, and means that needs are not being met.

What can we do with resentment? Here are some ideas:

» Be mindful of the feeling, step back and observe it, and name it.

» Notice thoughts and consider whether they are true, whether there is evidence for them (or not) or whether a different perspective can be found.

» Aim to defuse the feeling and let it pass like the weather (see p. 151).

» Know your triggers from past experiences (such as people not helping out or giving excuses).

» Be aware of your own expectations and perfectionism (see Chapter 6) if present and decide if you need to adjust your thinking.

» Do you need to bring in acceptance, such as when taking on a carer role (plus self-care) or forgiveness (when a genuine mistake has been made or hurt caused)?

» We all need to feel heard, so work on communication — your own and within relationships or families (see Chapter 9).

» Be compassionate towards yourself and empathetic to others.

» Practise saying no and learn assertiveness skills (see later in the chapter).

» If you are in an abusive situation, seeking help to ensure safety and to make decisions about the best way forward is vital, such as considering leaving the situation.

Strategies to manage resentment: Name the feeling and identify related thoughts, and check whether they are true. You may need to address issues in relationships, and practise saying no.

Boundaries

Let's talk about boundaries that refer to a limit or space between us and another person.[2] Setting healthy boundaries is a part of looking after our physical and mental health and wellbeing, and developing our sense of self. Research has shown that setting boundaries can have a positive effect on our emotional wellbeing, and learning how to say no has a positive effect on mental health.[3]

Boundaries involve a space between us and others, and setting limits.

Boundaries may be physical or emotional, and are part of our self-care and self-compassion, and sometimes self-protection. Here are a couple of examples:

> Nurul was going through a really busy time with work. Her friend Isabelle rang and said, 'We haven't seen each other for such a long time, how about I drop in on Friday night and bring takeaway and we can watch a movie together?' Nurul attempted to say that she'd prefer to take a rain check for a few weeks, but Isabelle insisted and Nurul felt she had to go along with the request, even though she had planned an early night.

> Anita was working for the family business and was being asked to do more and more tasks. She was feeling stressed and overwhelmed most of the time. Her manager (also her uncle) asked her to take on

an additional project. When she said that she had a full workload, her uncle said to her, 'That's fine for you, but the rest of us are doing our bit for the family and keeping the business afloat.' Anita felt she had to take on more but had no idea how she would manage the new task.

At times it is hard to set reasonable boundaries with others. One reason for this is being empathetic and not wanting to upset others. Plus we have often been trained to be people-pleasers (see p. 21). Past trauma or abuse can also lead to struggles to set boundaries, because they have previously been ignored by perpetrators. The net result is struggling to let friends, family, work colleagues or others know our limits and giving in to their requests and demands, which potentially drains or hurts us.

Here are some strategies that might help:

» Identify your current boundaries and whom they are with. Are there unhealthy boundaries with particular people?

» Reflect on times when you did not feel empowered to set a boundary, and on what got in the way (perhaps the actions of others, or your own thoughts).

» Consider any patterns of behaviour that have previously helped with setting boundaries or gotten in the way.

» Remember that we all have rights to set healthy boundaries.

» Practise saying no in a gracious but firm way, and give minimal or no explanation. Say it once and then move the conversation along. If you drop the subject, the other person is more likely to drop it, too!

» Sometimes we need to say more, as we need to let the other person know possible consequences. An example might be if a woman's partner insists that a large loan be taken out in both names, but the woman is not comfortable about the size of the loan. The consequence might be seeking financial advice or keeping finances separate.

» We all have a right to privacy, and boundaries often need to be set in relation to this.

» We may need to develop boundaries in relation to sexual practices and what we are comfortable with.

Set healthy boundaries: There are many ways to set boundaries, starting with recognizing that we have rights in relation to them. Practise strategies to set healthy ones.

Anger

We all feel angry at times, ranging in intensity from irritation to rage. Sometimes we express it in healthy ways, and sometimes in unhelpful behaviours. In this section, we will look at understanding and managing our own anger. Later on, in Chapter 10, we will explore intimate partner violence.

Anger is often related to something getting in the way of a desired outcome or when we believe there's a challenge to the way things 'should be'. Brené Brown describes it as an action emotion, that is, 'we want to do something when we feel it and were on the receiving end of it'.[4] It is important to acknowledge and understand anger, and learn ways to tame it at times.

Anger can be a normal, healthy reaction to feeling threatened and is part of our fight, flight or freeze (or survival) response. It can also follow on from feeling scared, sad, hurt, insecure or lonely. Anger can also occur when there is co-existing depression or substance use. Other factors that can contribute to anger are stress, frustration, being tired, hungry or in pain, shame, grief or physical withdrawal from certain drugs.

Anger changes the brain. It activates the nervous system and can change our thoughts and actions. Remember the limbic system in the brain, which houses the amygdala or emotional centre (see p. 46)? This part of the brain registers something like fear or rejection and triggers the fight, flight or freeze response, releasing loads of stress hormones into the body. These reduce activity in the brain cortex, which is responsible for making decisions and judgment. This is why it can be hard to make good decisions when feeling angry.

Anger can range from irritation to rage. It is often related to something getting in the way of the outcome we want or the way things 'should be'.

As mentioned, anger can range from feeling frustrated or annoyed to full-blown rage. On the one hand we want to recognise and allow ourselves to feel angry, but we don't want to take unreasonable or violent actions (because we are not thinking clearly). Anger becomes a problem when it impacts negatively on relationships, work and health or causes issues with the law. Here is an example:

> Roslyn struggled with anger at times. She had grown up with a very dominant father who would become angry and often rejected Ros at these times. Her first significant relationship was emotionally and physically abusive. Her second marriage was generally calm but her husband, Bob, would withdraw after an argument and Ros perceived this as rejection. She would become angry and at times Ros would yell loudly at him as she followed him around the house. Their pattern of behaviour was becoming more frequent, and upsetting, and they decided to seek relationship counselling.

Potential benefits of learning to manage anger are improved health and wellbeing, reduced risk of harm to oneself and others, increased self-confidence, improved relationships and better quality of life. Anger will always be one of our feelings, so it is not a matter of getting rid of it but changing how we use it and outgrowing any unhelpful behaviours.

Signs that anger is a problem include feeling angry a great deal of the time, anger being out of proportion to the triggering event or lasting a long time, and others saying that they are worried about your anger. Important signs are that the anger involves abusive behaviours, or is leading to problems in relationships or at work, or is causing mental health problems such as anxiety, depression or substance-related issues.

If these signs are evident, such as with Ros and Bob, it is important to take responsibility for them, despite shame often being present. It is the first step in dealing with anger issues, and deciding to get help is the next big step. Reaching out can be hard as it means making ourselves vulnerable. But it is better to reach out early, rather than when there has been a crisis.

It can help to heed psychiatrist Viktor Frankl's words: 'between stimulus and response there is a space. In that space is our power to choose our response. In our response lies our growth and our freedom.'[5] Stepping back and getting to know this space, and taking an alternative action can assist.

> Roslyn and Bob learnt to take some time apart before talking more about their disagreements. Bob worked on withdrawing less and as Roslyn understood her anger more, she learnt to soothe herself when triggered by rejection.

There are many strategies to help with taming anger. Not all will fit, but see which ones might assist you:

>> Understand the anger (maybe through talking or writing about it).

>> Use your journal to note both when the anger is occurring and any triggers.

>> Name any related feelings, such as hurt or shame. Then you need to deal with them via working with your thoughts and emotions (more on this later in the chapter).

>> Take responsibility for changing unhealthy behaviours.

» Let go of the idea that you can control other people.

» Identify signs of anger (e.g. breathing more quickly, feeling tense in the muscles). Then say 'Stop!' loudly in your mind, and count to 20 before responding.

» Take some time out to feel calmer.

» Only express anger in a way that fits with who you want to be.

» Look at other ways to express anger (such as exercise).

» Use distraction, such as listening to music or doing household tasks.

Here are some more ideas to consider:

» Do some regular relaxation or mindfulness (see Chapter 4).

» Review your boundaries or limits (your own and other people's).

» Communicate about the issues (listen and ask questions).

» Use problem-solving to sort out issues.

» When angry, delay speaking until you feel calmer.

» Develop helpful self-talk (e.g. 'stay calm, relax and breathe easy; I can do this').

» Develop empathy by working on understanding the other person's viewpoint.

» Don't sweat the small stuff! Instead ask, 'How important is this? Is it worth getting angry about?'

» Use humour to reduce the tension.

» Work on forgiving others more often.

Ways to tame anger: You can tame anger by understanding it and expressing it in ways that fit with who you want to be. Mindfulness, distraction, delaying strategies and reasonable self-talk can assist.

In terms of anger and thinking, it can also be useful to identify anger triggers. Reflect on thoughts prior to the anger, such as 'Bob stopped talking and shut down'. And consider related thoughts: 'He always does this, he doesn't love me any more'; feelings such as hurt or rejection; and on the related behaviours, such as 'I kept yelling at him'. Consider what would be more helpful, such as breathing or counting, and what fits with who you want to be.

Watch out for thinking traps (especially black-and-white thinking, mind-reading or labelling). Work on identifying them and challenging them. Unhelpful underlying beliefs can also be drivers of anger (such as 'it's not fair'). All the strategies covered earlier in the chapter can help. Detaching from our thoughts with mindfulness, or learning to sit with anger and defuse it, can be helpful (see p. 108).

Assertiveness

It can be life-changing to learn the difference between being assertive and being angry, and how to be more assertive. Assertiveness means clearly communicating our view or needs, without becoming aggressive. It involves respecting ourselves and others. It can involve changing the ways in which we relate to people and the behaviours that we use.

Being more assertive can be helpful in many situations, such as dealing with annoyances, responding to criticism or turning down requests.

Let's take an example in which we feel our rights are not being taken into account at work. Maybe a colleague is talking over us at meetings and not asking for our views on a task we know a lot about. Assertiveness can help us express our feelings about their behaviours. It is good to acknowledge the other person first by saying something like, 'I appreciate this is a challenging situation,' and then we can go on to use what we call an 'I' statement in a calm and steady way.

This statement sounds like this:

» 'I feel ...' (name the feeling)

» 'When you ...' (state what the unacceptable behaviour is in a non-blaming way)

» 'Because ...' (explain the effects of the behaviour on you)

» 'I'd prefer ...' (what you would like to happen).[6]

Using this as a guide, the work example might then sound like: 'I appreciate this is a challenging situation. I feel disappointed when you don't ask my views on it because I have a lot of knowledge about the area. I'd prefer it if I could have the opportunity to share my views.'

Loneliness

Loneliness relates to feeling disconnected or isolated from others. As humans, we need social connections and meaningful interactions, just as we need water and food. Belonging to and being accepted by a group helps us to survive and thrive in life, and our physical and mental health are impacted without them. In particular, loneliness has been shown to increase inflammation in the body and decrease our cognitive function. It is also associated with depression and anxiety.[7]

Loneliness can affect all of us, briefly or in the longer term. Loneliness is one of the reasons COVID-19 lockdowns and isolation periods had such an impact on us. Young adults and older adults are more at risk from loneliness. Peer acceptance and establishing identity are so important to young people, and older people may lose partners, or family members may be busy with their own lives.

We might also be more vulnerable to loneliness depending on our personality traits (which may or may not help us connect with other people), our attachment style (more on attachment in Chapter 9), our work and socio-economic and educational status, education level, and whether we are living alone or in a relationship. We can feel lonely in a relationship if there is not meaningful connection.

Loneliness can affect all of us, and may impact our physical and mental health. Investing in key relationships is important.

Loneliness may not be acknowledged as an issue by others, because it is assumed we all have to deal with it at times. However, it is an issue that impacts our self-worth and causes distress including sadness or shame, and it is now seen as a major health issue. As mentioned earlier, some countries are appointing ministers for loneliness to address the issue at a society level. We are more connected than ever digitally, but the question is whether we have 'real world' interactions or not.[8]

In relation to individuals, we need to address both building social connections and working with our thoughts, feelings and behaviours.

The following strategies may assist:

> » Remember loneliness is a feeling, not necessarily a fact!
>
> » Loneliness can trigger negative thinking, such as 'they don't want to see me', so watch out for this and challenge any unhelpful thoughts.
>
> » Build on existing relationships with family, friends or neighbours.
>
> » Take action and phone or visit family members when possible.
>
> » Connect (phone, email, meet up) with friends or work colleagues.
>
> » Head out to places with people, such as the beach or a shopping centre, and have some contact by saying hello and having a chat with shop assistants.
>
> » Take up a hobby or take a class, or join a group.
>
> » Focus on the needs or others (such as through volunteering).
>
> » Listen to the radio, including talkback radio. Think about phoning in!
>
> » Call a support service or help line.

One of the main messages about loneliness from clinical psychologist and loneliness expert, Dr Michelle Lim, is that it is the quality and not the number or quantity of our connections that is so influential. We need to invest our time and energy into quality relationships wherever possible.

Reducing loneliness: Connecting with others is important, as is focusing on 'quality, not quantity' of relationships.

Rejection

There is no doubt we have all experienced rejection at some stage, whether from family, a friend, a potential or established intimate partner, our workplace or via social media. Rejection is the action of pushing someone away, and it may trigger feelings of stress, shame, sadness or grief. Bullying is in part an act of rejection. Rejection goes against our innate need to connect and belong.[9]

Romantic rejection is hard to deal with, especially when it comes as a shock or is carried out in an insensitive way, such as news delivered by text or email rather than in person. It can trigger hurt and anger, and thoughts about it being our fault or not being enough. It feels pretty awful and reduces our ability to think clearly.

Research has shown that the brain responds to social pain in a way that is similar to physical pain. The same areas of the brain are activated. It does hurt. The psychological effects of rejection may include trauma and depression. It can also play a significant role in anxiety (including social anxiety), and those with borderline personality disorder are highly sensitive to it.[10]

Rejection activates the same areas of the brain as physical pain. We need to learn to soothe the pain.

So how do we manage feelings of rejection? Processing this emotion takes time. We need to soothe the emotional pain (see tolerating distress skills in Chapter 7), manage any related anger (see earlier in this chapter) and work on our self-belief by quitting negative self-talk (see Chapter 3). Processing earlier traumas may also assist (see Chapter 10).

Sometimes we also need to find a different perspective, consider whether we need to change any of our behaviours, and search for any positives that may come from the rejection. Seeking support from our circle or talking with a therapist can help.

Tolerating emotional distress

In this chapter and in Chapter 4, we have looked at a number of emotions that feel uncomfortable and can create distress. Having the skills to cope with these emotions and soothe ourselves is vital. We have looked at various approaches in previous chapters, but let's explore another valuable one.

Psychiatrist Dr Marsha Linehan developed **Dialectical Behaviour Therapy**. It stems from the idea that we are all doing our best to manage, even if we are engaging in an unhelpful behavior. The use of the word 'dialectical' refers to acceptance of self, at the same time as recognizing the need for change. This enables us to accept we are doing our best while also aiming for changes in our behaviours and how we manage emotions.

Originally developed to assist clients to manage symptoms related to borderline personality disorder, Dialectical Behaviour Therapy is particularly useful if there is a struggle with strong emotions or a tendency to react more intensely to a situation than others. However, many of the ideas and skills from this therapy are valuable for all of us in managing life's challenges and distressing emotions. It has also been found to be effective with a range of mental health issues, including depression, eating disorders, substance-related issues and post-traumatic stress disorder.

We are all doing our best to manage. If we can accept ourselves, but also recognize the need for change, we can begin to heal.

This approach suggests that we have:

1. the 'emotion mind', which acts when feelings are in the driver's seat and controlling our thoughts and actions (e.g. acting impulsively)

2. the 'reasonable mind', which focuses on logic and ignores feelings

3. the 'wise mind', which balances both, recognizing and respecting feelings, but reacting in a reasonable, logical way.[11]

We might recognize these parts of our mind if we think about how we have responded to different experiences in life. An example would be a situation where we have been criticized. Our 'emotion mind' might have responded with anger or disappointment, whereas our 'reasonable mind' might have recalled events that triggered the criticism. The 'wise mind' steps back to observe the situation and our thoughts and feelings, so that we can respond in a considered way. Perhaps write down a few thoughts about recognizing the wise mind in your journal.

Dialectical Behaviour Therapy acknowledges that we often want a better life, and that we need many skills to achieve this. Time is spent reflecting on values and living consistently with these to build self-worth and meaning. It also incorporates taking action aligned with our values, and encourages us to connect with valued people, work or spiritual pursuits (if relevant to us).

This therapy incorporates many useful ideas and skills related to:

» mindfulness

» distress tolerance

» emotion regulation

» interpersonal effectiveness

» behavioural skills.

Mindfulness skills form the foundation for the approach, and mindfulness meditations and breathing are encouraged (see p. 92). Mindful observation of emotions and behaviours is utilized in many of the skills and helps to activate our wise mind.

In relation to tolerating distress and soothing or regulating emotions, this therapy adopts the idea that the more we struggle with and try to avoid distress, the worse it often becomes. At times we cannot change situations that trigger distress, and we need to work on acceptance or being willing to experience a situation as it is in the moment and without judgment (that is, mindfully).

Let's unpack this a little more. The term 'radical acceptance' is sometimes used and refers to practising acceptance even if our feelings are painful, knowing that the situation or the feelings are not how we want things to be. We hold the feelings mindfully (like holding a baby), without expectations of change. However, sometimes the unexpected or change does follow, especially when we utilize our skills.[12]

When feeling emotional distress, we may need to relax (such as using relaxation skills) and rest. Or we can use distraction from the uncomfortable feelings via daily activities (such as household tasks), exercise, patting a pet, gardening or watching a film. We can come up with a list of pleasant activities that soothe us, such as having a bath, reading a book or listening to music, and turn to these when feeling distressed. Using the various senses may help, such as looking at nature, smelling the fresh air or tasting a soothing tea. It can help to focus outside of ourselves on someone or something else.

To tolerate distressing emotions: We can soothe ourselves with relaxation, distraction or pleasant activities.

We can also create a 'distress tolerance box', decorate it and fill it with activities that help soothe us, such as favourite photos, quotes, prayers if you like, or an aromatherapy candle. Visualizations of a place in which we feel safe (such as a cottage or the beach) can also help, and we can focus on other thoughts (counting to ten, saying the letters of the alphabet, reading a book).

Self-care and regular routines are seen as part of regulating emotions, as eating well, avoiding harmful substances, getting regular exercise and getting enough sleep all help. HALT is a great acronym that stands for Hungry, Angry, Lonely and Tired. This is when we are more vulnerable to distress and unhelpful behaviours, and it acts as a reminder to address these factors. We also need to plan for triggers for problem behaviours and have strategies ready to go, such as using our self-soothing skills or more helpful self-talk.[13]

Dialectical Behaviour Therapy includes education about emotions (see Chapter 2) and encourages recognition and naming of emotions. It links emotions to healthy and unhealthy behaviours. Self-harming behaviors fall into the latter, and will be considered in the next section. It also adopts the idea of doing something that will create an opposite emotion (if anxious, listen to calming music; if sad, watching a comedy), and also pushing negative thoughts away (writing them on a piece of paper, then crumpling up the paper and throwing it away) or focusing on a pleasant memory instead.

Another practical strategy to use when emotions are distressing is STOPP. This was covered earlier, but let's take another look. It involves taking a 'helicopter view' of emotions:

> » **S** for stopping and pausing, not acting immediately.
> » **T** for taking a step back (look at things as if through a window or different lens) and breathing.
> » **O** for observing what is going on around you, and your thoughts and feelings. Identify your self-talk and ask whether it is helpful.
> » **P** is putting in some perspective by seeing the situation as an outside observer and considering what they would make of it.
> » **P** is also for proceeding mindfully, practising what works you, and doing what is appropriate and most helpful (using the wise mind).[14]

Other strategies to tolerate distress: Self-care, a distress tolerance box, doing the opposite, sitting with emotion or the STOPP technique can help.

We have already talked about emotions and actions being closely linked. Dialectical Behaviour Therapy says every emotion triggers an 'action urge'. When we are anxious, the urge is to avoid. When we are sad, we stop doing things and withdraw. When there is shame, the urge is to defend ourselves or hide, and when we are angry the urge is to fight.[15]

The problem is that these urges can cause more problems, and so one strategy is to take the opposite action! This involves choosing an urge to work on, and think about, our voice, posture, words and actions we use when acting on the urge. Then we identify the opposite action (i.e. how to change our voice, posture, words and actions to carry this out), and commit to the opposite action in situations that trigger the urge. Examples include:

» When anxious, approach what is feared and do what you have been avoiding, stand tall and speak quietly.

» When sad, be more active, get involved, stand straight and speak in a strong voice.

» When angry, validate the other person, adopt a relaxed posture and speak softly.

Dialectical Behaviour Therapy also suggests using problem-solving skills in relation to emotions and perhaps the results of action urges.

It involves looking at our thoughts, feelings and actions at each stage of the event and considering what we could have done differently, such as using coping skills or opposite actions. Finally, it teaches interpersonal skills such as listening to and validating others, dealing with conflict (see Chapter 9), recognizing our rights and boundaries in a relationship, and developing assertiveness skills (see earlier this chapter). Social media skills may also be addressed, such as not saying anything negative and not reacting to negative comments.

Once the approach is understood, and the skills taught, the final step is much practice. We can do this through exposure in our minds (visualizing a recent emotionally triggering experience, scoring the emotion from 0 to 10 and shutting the scene off somewhere between 4 and 5). Then practise using our skills. This can be repeated, plus we can practise the skills in real life when we feel ready.[16]

Self-harm and suicidality

This section explores **non-suicidal self-harm** (behaviours deliberately hurting the body, such as cutting) and **suicidal behaviours**. It offers information and strategies to assist the person and their family or carers, but these do not replace emergency support or professional assistance. So, if struggling, please don't wait — seek help straight away.

Overall, between 1–2 per cent of deaths are by suicide, and every year a significant number of suicide deaths occur worldwide with over 3000 each year in Australia, 47,000 in the United States and 6000 in the United Kingdom (the rate of death by suicide in women compared to men is one to three).[17,18] Non-suicidal self-injuring behaviours have become increasingly common in adolescence and young adulthood — the rate in adolescence is about 17 per cent; the rate in adults reduces significantly to about 5–6 per cent.[19]

At the centre of all crises is suffering and extremely distressing emotions. Suicidal thoughts and behaviours may be motivated by the desire to escape or relieve distressing feelings or situations, or to communicate feelings or change how other people are responding.[20] The reasons for the self-injuring behaviours often relate to managing, painful or overwhelming feelings, self-punishment or as a way of communicating the emotional pain with others.

Wanting to relieve distress or escape suffering may motivate non-suicidal self-harm or suicidal behaviours.

Experiencing non-suicidal self-harm or suicidal thoughts or behaviours is very distressing, but please know that there is always hope, as whatever the situation may be, it can improve. We all have many strengths and resources within us to draw on and support and help are available.

Non-suicidal self-harm

Inflicting damage to one's own body without the intention of suicide (and not consistent with cultural norms) is known as non-suicidal self-harm.[21] Mental health issues, such as mood or anxiety disorders, eating disorders or borderline personality disorders (see p. 299) are risk factors, along with struggles in regulating emotions or high levels of self-criticism. Trauma, social isolation, family problems, gender identity or sexuality issues and substance-related problems are also risk factors.

The most common methods of non-suicidal self-harm are cutting or scratching, deliberately hitting the body on a hard surface, punching, hitting or slapping yourself, and biting or burning. The brain learns that physical pain leads to less emotional pain, and so the behaviours are reinforced and keep occurring.

There is emotional pain, and the brain learns that physical pain reduces the emotional pain, reinforcing the behaviours.

Mental health first aid

First of all, it is important not to assume that those who self-harm are suicidal, and also not to presume they are not feeling suicidal. Studies have shown that 10 per cent of people who had injured themselves in the past four weeks had made a suicide attempt in the last year, and 60 per cent had thoughts of suicide.[22]

The only way to know if someone is having suicidal thoughts is to ask them. If you suspect someone is self-harming, discuss it with them if you are able to, in a private place. You might say something like, 'Sometimes when people are in a lot of emotional pain, they injure themselves on purpose. Is that how your injury happened?'

If you interrupt someone who is self-injuring, stay as calm as possible and intervene in a supportive and non-judgmental way. You can say that you are concerned and ask them if you can provide support. You can assist them by expressing empathy, listening to them, validating their feelings or concerns, and giving support and reassurance that there is help available.

It is important not to promise to keep the behaviour a secret, and to encourage the person to seek professional help (from a doctor or mental health professional), and assist them to do so if they ask. You might need to organize medical help (to check wounds) if needed.

If the self-harm is severe, interfering with functioning, or if the person has injured their eyes or genitals, or expressed a desire to die, contact the emergency services immediately.

Know when to seek help: Self-harming behaviours can be severe and result in significant injuries. If this is the case, it is important to seek help urgently.

Seeing a therapist

When someone who has been self-harming seeks help from a therapist, they will focus on increasing healthy coping skills rather than removing unhealthy ones. This will involve learning self-soothing and ways to regulate emotions that were outlined earlier in the chapter, as well as strategies to effectively communicate their needs.

Therapists will talk about alternatives to self-harming behaviour, such as speaking to someone (family, friend, helpline), and delaying the behaviour (feelings come and go, so any urge to self-harm will also pass). We can wait five minutes, then wait another five minutes more;

count from one to 100 or do some breathing exercises (see Chapter 4).

It is important to make the environment safe (such as making sure that sharp objects are removed), or we can go to a different spot in the house or change the environment by going out into the garden. Distraction can help, such as watching a film or doing some exercise. Having a self-harm distraction box containing things to focus on (such as music or soothing aromatherapy) can help.

Dealing with urges to self-harm: An urge is a feeling, and all feelings come and go. Delaying self-harm, using distraction or soothing activities such as watching a movie can help.

If the behaviours are punishing, then learning self-compassion is important (see p. 49). If anger is present, talking about it with a trusted person or punching a punching bag might help. Some of the strategies included earlier in the chapter may also help reduce anger. Other ways of reducing self-harm include doing an alternative activity, such as holding a piece of ice (it is distracting and there is some discomfort involved), having a cry or writing in the journal.

About suicidality

We have already mentioned some of the statistics about suicide. Being aware of the risk factors is important, as ultimately we aim to detect suicidal feeling and thoughts early and intervene. We also want to enhance our protective factors, which include feeling mentally healthy with a strong sense of wellbeing, treating any mental health issues, aiming for social connection, a sense of purpose, employment and financial security.

Risk factors for suicidal behaviours include previous suicide attempts, mental health issues or a recent discharge from a psychiatric hospital. Physical illness, especially if terminal, painful or debilitating is also a risk factor, as is a family history of suicide or substance-related or mental health issues. Rejection by a significant person and relationship breakdown and divorce are risk factors.

Other risk factors include a history of bullying, trauma or abuse, being socially isolated, a tendency to take risks or be impulsive, recent exposure to the suicide of someone else, loss and grief, family problems, unemployment or any changes to employment or poverty. A significant risk factor is a sense of hopelessness, particularly from social issues or depression.

Indigenous women and individuals identifying as gay, transsexual or with another gender or sexual identity are at a higher risk.[23,24]

Suicide prevention

There is a range of suicide prevention strategies, including:

> » mental health first aid (just like a physical injury, a mental health crisis, such as suicidal thinking, requires first aid)
> » having access to information
> » reaching out for individual help
> » help for the family.

Mental health first aid training and resources help us to offer assistance to the person experiencing suicidal thoughts before they are able to access professional help. If concerned about risk of suicide, we can watch for these signals or warning signs:

>> Threats of suicide, searching for ways to kill themselves (such as online searches, looking for weapons), talking about death or suicide, or normalizing it as a way to deal with their current situation.

>> Expressing hopelessness, anger, revenge seeking and acting recklessly or using substances.

>> Saying they are trapped or there is 'no way out', or that there is no reason for living or no sense of purpose in life.

>> Withdrawal from family or friends (or making uncharacteristic contact).

>> Signs of anxiety or depression such as agitation, inability to sleep or dramatic changes in mood (including a sudden improvement in mood or calmness).

If we are concerned about suicidality, we can say that we are worried, and that we care. Expressing empathy for them and what they are going through can help. It is best to talk in a matter-of-fact way and ask directly whether they are suicidal ('Are you having thoughts of suicide? Are you thinking about killing yourself?'). Let them know suicidal thoughts are common and can be associated with treatable mental health issues, and advise them to get help and offer to assist with this, such as calling a crisis service.[25]

If we think the person might be at the point of ending their life, indicated by them saying they have decided how or when to kill themselves, that they have access to the means to take their life, or that they are more at risk due to past behaviours or substance use, ***do not*** leave them alone and call the emergency services.

To help a person who is suicidal: Do not leave them alone, and assist them to get help (call emergency services).

Reaching out for help

When there are suicidal thoughts or there have been suicidal behaviours, it is important to seek help. Depending on the issues, help may be sought from emergency services, crisis or mental health services or a doctor or therapist. The most important thing is to feel safe and have the opportunity to talk.

Suicidal thoughts or behaviours are often very distressing (they can be frightening and associated with a sense of shame), so there will be relief at being able to talk about what is happening.

Doctors and mental health professionals will assess the degree of risk with the aim of differentiating low risk versus high risk of attempting suicide, and they will manage any risk so that help can be provided to stave off suicide attempts. They will take into account risk factors and protective factors (such as family support) and check out thoughts about suicide and how long these have been present (e.g. any threats, plans or preparations, recent or past suicidal behaviours).

Health professionals will also investigate any mental health issues, level of functioning day to day, any substance use, social supports or other resources. The level of care that is needed will be considered, such as managing with some phone support, or care provided by family and a local doctor. A safety plan may be helpful for individuals. This involves writing a plan when feeling calm and writing about warning signs of a crisis, creating a safe place, people who can be contacted as well as professional help.

As risk increases more support is needed, from mental health services, a therapist or psychiatrist. Sometimes an immediate referral to a hospital for further assessment, and possibly admission to ensure safety, may be needed.

What happens in therapy?

When individual treatment is needed, it will focus on providing support and listening, and developing self-awareness of thoughts and feelings. Suicidal thinking or behaviours may be attempts to solve problems that seem intolerable, and so problem-solving any worrying issues and learning new problem-solving skills may be helpful (see Chapter 4).

Dealing with unhelpful thoughts or underlying beliefs through Cognitive Behaviour Therapy is vital (see p. 69). The following strategy for dealing with suicidal thoughts may be helpful:

> We actually have 'suicidal thoughts' rather than 'feeling suicidal' (the feeling may be depression, anger or despair). Often these thoughts are really distressing and overwhelming, but it is important to recognize that they are thoughts only and may not be based on truth. It is important to notice the thoughts and to understand that they may be driven by depressed mood or recent events, and to know that we can deal with the thoughts in different ways. We can challenge them ('Am I catastrophizing the situation, or seeing it more bleakly than it is? Is there another way to think about things?'), or we can observe them and let them pass.

A therapist can provide some guidance on how to deal with uncomfortable emotions, such as anger, guilt or shame, and ways to tolerate distress. They may introduce a principle from Dialectical Behaviour Therapy that we can have opposing thoughts and motivations (e.g. a desire to end life but to also seek help and live). The therapy builds on the desire to live and the reasons for this.

A therapist can also provide assistance with any interpersonal issues, such as conflict, relationship breakdown or bullying, and loss and grief counselling if relevant. Identifying our resources and strengths can be very useful, as we can use these strengths to assist with coping.

Family members affected by a person's suicidal thinking or behaviours also need support and assistance. Seeking help from a doctor is a good place to start. They can provide support and assistance, as well as organize a referral to a therapist if needed. If the person has been harmed or has died, there will be significant trauma and many distressing emotions. Assistance will most likely be needed, so again, please seek some support and help.

Let's summarize

Resentment and anger have been explored in this chapter. It is important to address them as they cause distress and can interfere with work, relationships and our health and wellbeing. We looked at two important strategies to manage these emotions, namely boundaries and assertiveness. These can be life-changing.

We also considered loneliness and rejection. Loneliness is a worldwide health concern and is known to have very significant impacts on our mental health and wellbeing. The key is the quality rather than the quantity of our relationships.

We then explored ways to tolerate emotional distress, drawing in particular on Dialectical Behaviour Therapy. This recognizes that we are doing our best to manage, but can also recognize the need for change. It introduces our 'wise mind', which can help us find a balance between our 'emotion mind' and our 'reasonable mind'. This approach also teaches many skills in tolerating distress and regulating emotion.

Importantly, in this chapter we talked about non-suicidal self-harm and suicidal behaviours. A mental health first aid approach was described, along with some practical coping strategies. Reaching out for help is vital.

It is also important to keep the focus on prevention as individuals and as communities, by working towards improved mental health and wellbeing and flourishing. The keys that may assist are summarized here:

» To manage resentment, name the feeling and identify related thoughts and check whether they are true. Address any relationship issues and practise saying no.

» Set healthy boundaries.

» Tame anger by understanding it and expressing it in ways that fit with who you want to be. Mindfulness, distraction, delaying strategies and reasonable self-talk can assist.

» Reduce loneliness by connecting with others, focusing on 'quality, not quantity' of relationships.

» To tolerate distressing emotion, you can soothe yourself with relaxation, distraction or pleasant activities.

» Other strategies to tolerate distress: self-care, a distress tolerance box, doing the opposite, sitting with emotion or the STOPP technique.

» Know when to seek help: Self-harming behaviours can be severe and result in significant injuries. If this is the case, is important to seek help urgently.

» Dealing with urges to self-harm: An urge is a feeling, and all feelings come and go. Delaying self-harm, using distraction or soothing activities such as watching a movie can help.

» To help a person who is suicidal: Do not leave them alone, and assist them to get help (call emergency services).

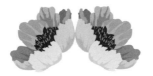

DEALING WITH ISSUES ACROSS THE LIFESPAN

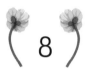

8

Managing menopause, hormonal and reproductive issues

"

Courage, Dear Heart

— C.S. Lewis

This chapter focuses on a number of the transitions in life related to our reproductive and hormonal functions. These times are also marked by other changes, such as becoming a parent or the end of menstruation and our ability to reproduce. To set the scene, we will cover background information about the menstrual cycle and hormones, and their impact on mood.

Some women have very few issues over the years with menstruation, pregnancy and post-birth, or menopause. Other women experience a range of struggles and are sometimes impacted hugely by these transitions. For these reasons we are going to explore mental health issues related to the menstrual cycle, pregnancy and birth, and also around menopause.

Unfortunately, we are not able to look at all of the important topics related to reproduction and hormones, but we will consider the ones mentioned and also miscarriage, stillbirth and infertility. Our focus will be on the psychological and social impacts of these issues, and ways to manage the related distress.

About the menstrual cycle, hormones and mood

It is thought that hormonal changes related to our reproductive systems play a role in our increased risk of depression and depressive episodes in bipolar disorder. In this section we will cover some background information about the menstrual cycle, as well as the interaction between hormones and mood.

The menstrual cycle begins at menarche or the first period, often around twelve or thirteen years of age, and ends with menopause or the final period, on average at 51 or 52 years old (but ranging from 45 to 55 years old). Every woman's cycle is unique and individual, and cycles vary in timing and heaviness across the lifespan.[1]

Every woman's cycle is unique and will vary across the lifespan.

The role of the menstrual cycle is to prepare the body for pregnancy.

This leads to the development and release of an egg from the ovary (ovulation) and growth of the internal lining of the uterus, to prepare it for pregnancy. When a pregnancy does not occur, a period results. The menstrual cycle occurs because of a complex relationship between hormones from the brain and the ovaries. Oestrogen and progesterone are the main hormones involved in the cycle, but there are a number of others. We also have testosterone.

A woman's menstrual cycle is divided into four phases, namely the menstrual phase (period), follicular phase (development of egg-containing follicles), ovulation phase (egg released) and luteal phase (post-ovulation). The maturing follicle leads to a surge in oestrogen that prepares the uterus to receive the egg. Progesterone rises in the second half of the cycle to help maintain an egg if it is fertilized. If the egg isn't fertilized it dies, and the levels of oestrogen and progesterone drop.[2]

Oral contraceptives and mood

We have been using oral contraceptives since the 1960s. These contain artificial oestrogen such as ethinylestradiol and progestogens, or progestogens alone. In general, oestrogen seems to be protective of brain functioning, including our thinking and memory, and also our ability to regulate emotions. For some women progesterone negatively impacts brain function.

These hormones influence our brain cells, possibly via the different brain neurotransmitters or messengers and their receptors (which transmit the messengers into the cells). These messengers include serotonin, dopamine and gamma aminobutyric acid. As mentioned earlier, we don't fully understand these influences, and it may depend on related substances such as enzymes (which influence chemical reactions) and what is happening at the cellular level.

It has been found that many women experience mood changes when on the oral contraceptive pill, especially young women.[3] This may be related to the amounts or type of oestrogen and progesterone contained in the particular pill (particularly synthetic progesterone). There is also variation between women as to sensitivity to various hormones. This is why, when starting the pill or any other hormonal treatment, a comprehensive assessment, including past history of depressed mood, needs to be done and an individualised approach taken. Seeing a doctor with a specific interest in women's health may assist. There is also a range of alternate forms of contraception that can be considered, or that may need to be considered.

In the next section we will look at mental health issues that may occur at different times during our lives, including premenstrually, around the birth of a baby and around menopause. More discussion about the influence of hormones on mood at these times will be included.

Premenstrual syndrome and premenstrual dysphoric disorder

The majority of women (80 per cent) experience some changes physically, emotionally or cognitively (concentration, memory) associated with their menstrual cycles.[4] In fact, menstruation may be associated with several 'premenstrual syndromes' that can vary in intensity. They represent a spectrum of symptoms or conditions associated with the premenstrual phase of the cycle. During this phase oestrogen levels fall, and progesterone levels rise.

Menstruation may be associated with several 'premenstrual syndromes,' including premenstrual dysphoric disorder.

One is premenstrual syndrome, which occurs in the week (or two) before menstruation and improves after menstruation. This syndrome may involve symptoms such as bloating and headaches, and also irritability and disturbed mood. It is less severe than 'premenstrual dysphoric disorder', but still challenging to manage.

The other end of the spectrum is premenstrual dysphoric disorder, which is suffered by around 10 per cent of women. Symptoms are cyclical and include depressed mood (can be sudden and severe), mood swings, anxiety, tearfulness, poor concentration, lethargy and feeling overwhelmed. These symptoms often interfere with the ability to function at home, in relationships or at work.[5]

It is thought that these issues may have a basis in our genetics. Some differences in our biology have been found in women experiencing premenstrual dysphoric disorder, including changes in sleep patterns and various differences in hormones (such as thyroid and stress-related issues). These changes may contribute to being vulnerable to the disorder. A history of post-traumatic stress disorder may be associated with premenstrual dysphoric disorder, and may be related to the effects of trauma on the autonomic nervous system and our stress response (see p. 83).[6] However, the main risk factors for premenstrual dysphoric disorder are fluctuations in our hormones related to the menstrual cycle and the impact of these on the brain. For some women progesterone and its breakdown products can have a negative effect, particularly on anxiety symptoms. However, we vary in sensitivity to these effects.[7] We know, too, that having premenstrual dysphoric disorder can lead to greater risk of developing depression and anxiety. Equally, pre-existing depression or anxiety symptoms may be made worse during the premenstrual phase.

For all of these reasons, it is important that thorough physical and mental health checks are carried out, and that the symptoms are not overlooked or misdiagnosed for another cyclical mood problem. Careful assessment of the risk of self-harm and suicidal thoughts is vital. Treatment many involve adopting positive lifestyle measures (such as working on sleep and exercising) and therapy.

Complementary therapies include various vitamins and supplements. However, premenstrual dysphoric disorder often requires treatment with particular oral contraceptives (non-synthetic) and other hormonal therapies, or antidepressant medication may be used during the premenstrual period. There is currently research on newer drugs which impact gamma aminobutyric acid in particular.

Help is available: Various strategies can help relieve premenstrual symptoms, including working on sleep and using exercise. Cognitive Behaviour Therapy and various medications can assist.

Perinatal phase

Let's look at the perinatal phase or period, which includes pregnancy and the postnatal phase. Pregnancy is often a time of happiness and excitement. It is also a time of many changes related to the body, relationships and career, and potentially changes to our sense of identity and the future. Many women and their partners will navigate pregnancy and the transition into parenthood without significant distress, and the focus will be on maintaining physical and mental health and wellbeing. However, some will face challenges during this time.[8]

We are not going to focus on ways to generally maintain health and wellbeing during pregnancy as there are many good resources available. Many of the steps from Chapter 2 may also be helpful (see 'Ten steps towards mental health and wellbeing' on p. 31, and note that guidance from a health professional is needed with step 10). Instead, we are going to look at how to manage some of the challenges that may be associated with this time, and which impact women and their partners or families.

Some women may experience pregnancy with an existing mental disorder, or develop a mental health problem for the first time. Perinatal mental health issues affect people from all backgrounds and regardless of age, and anxiety and depression affect up to one in five women during pregnancy. There are a number of risk factors related to this, including unplanned pregnancy, history of mental health problems or substance-related issues, past or current abuse or trauma, past infertility or pregnancy complications, stressful life events or lack of support.[9] Remember, too, that intimate partner and family violence appears to be more prevalent in pregnancy and may be a major risk factor.

The perinatal period may be a time of great joy, but perinatal mental health issues can occur, especially anxiety or depression.

After delivery, some disruptions to mood can occur. The 'blues' might occur in the first week or so and can involve tearfulness and mood fluctuations. The blues are common and are thought to be related to fluctuations in various hormones. Issues with lack of social support and sleep deprivation may also contribute.

Postpartum or postnatal depression is less common and more severe, affecting up to 15 per cent of women (and 10 per cent of men). Many factors can contribute, and a past history of depression, especially related to hormonal influences (premenstrually or with the contraceptive pill) may increase vulnerability at this time.[10] Note that the COVID-19 pandemic has added more stress to this time in life, with partners or family unable to be present at births, for example.

It is important to identify if there is a problem with mood or anxiety, and this is why depression questionnaires are used routinely by family doctors, in maternity hospitals and at subsequent health checks in the community. If there are symptoms of depression, it is also vital that a physical health check is done, including blood tests to exclude physical causes such as thyroid problems or anaemia.

Support from family doctors and community midwives or child nurses can assist, as can psychological therapy. This involves working with any self-critical thoughts such as 'not being a good enough mother' or 'being a failure'. These thoughts are often related to high expectations about being a 'perfect mother', or being competent or in control all of the time. If we are not meeting these expectations, we can feel guilt or shame (see p. 160). The media and other societal influences often foster ideas about being the 'perfect mother'. However, being a parent is a challenging role, and being competent all of the time is not actually possible! In addition, we cannot be fully in control of everything when we have a baby. They have a way of ignoring control!

At this point, let's hear about Sophie and Maxie's story:

> Sophie and Maxie were expecting their first child and busily preparing. Sophie read every parenting book that she could, to learn about their new roles in life. Then the pandemic began. Sophie was told she would need to deliver alone and leave the hospital as soon as possible after the delivery. In her mind the birth had been planned, and this didn't fit with the plan. Sophie was devastated.
>
> When Sophie came home, baby Eleanor was unsettled. After a week Maxie had to go back to work and so Sophie managed most nights with the baby. Sophie's mother stepped in to help, but Sophie struggled with this. She so wanted to be the best mother, and blamed herself for 'failing'.
>
> At Eleanor's health check, the community nurse recognized that Sophie had been impacted by these events and heard her self-critical thoughts. She was supportive of Sophie and organized some other help.
>
> Maxie pulled back from work and they worked on ways for Sophie to get some more sleep. Sophie also started to see that the birth

had been very hard but that she had somehow gotten through. She also realised that her own expectations of herself were not realistic. Things were improving and Sophie and Maxie could relax and enjoy the baby more.

Drop the idea of being a perfect mother: This is not humanly possible, and we may need to challenge some of our thoughts or beliefs. The aim is less self-criticism and more self-compassion.

Assistance with postnatal depression or anxiety needs to be comprehensive and supportive and involve partners or family if possible. Increasing practical supports can be helpful, as can addressing sleep issues and relationship concerns. Having some time out from the practical tasks of parenthood is important, as well as focusing each day on something positive that has occurred.

Medications may be used if psychological assistance alone is not reducing the depression or anxiety. Note that in many ways the management of postnatal depression or anxiety is similar to managing depression or anxiety at other times, and much of the information provided in Chapters 4 and 6 will be relevant.

Postpartum psychosis is a less common issue but is very serious and considered a medical emergency. Mood fluctuations, symptoms of psychosis (such as delusional thinking or hallucinations) and confusion are common features. Urgent treatment is required, and this may involve hospital or medications, therapy and assistance with bonding or attaching to the baby.

At times the birth may be traumatic due to the nature of the labour or delivery, lack of support, a sense of lack of control or threat, as well as the medical procedures involved. Trauma may result in acute stress or post-traumatic stress disorder (see Chapter 10). This may be confused with the baby 'blues' or post-partum depression, but the background of trauma and the related symptoms, such as flashbacks or nightmares, differentiates it from these. Seeing a doctor or therapist experienced in this area is important, and there may be birth trauma support services locally.

Miscarriage and stillbirth, infertility and endometriosis

Unfortunately, millions of women worldwide experience miscarriage, stillbirth or infertility when wanting to conceive and have a baby. **Miscarriage** refers to the spontaneous expulsion from the uterus of the foetus and placenta before 20 weeks of gestation, and **stillbirth** refers to birth after this time, and when there are no signs of life.[11] These all involve significant loss and grief, and potentially trauma.[12] However, their impact has been under-recognized in the past.

Many women who experience miscarriage feel great distress. Unfortunately, many of the causes of miscarriage are not well understood, but there can be chromosomal abnormalities in the foetus. Most miscarriages cannot be prevented and the woman is not to blame. It is important to acknowledge the loss and grief and look to others for support.[13]

Recent studies have shown that women who miscarry can experience depression or anxiety which can continue for a number of years. Having a baby later does not necessarily resolve the mental health issues. Previous pregnancy loss is therefore a risk factor for postnatal depression.[14]

Stillbirth is extremely distressing and can also result in anxiety and depression.[15] Good care and support after the birth are vital. Symptoms can persist for a long time, and impact wellbeing and day-to-day ability to function.

Social support is important as is seeking therapy, as illustrated in Kristen and Suresh's story:

> Kristen and her partner Suresh saw a therapist together. Three months previously they had been excited about the birth of their first baby, but their little boy was stillborn. They were devastated. They spent time cuddling their son, named and dressed him, and there was a funeral. They were supporting each other in coping with their loss and their family was being very helpful. But they were experiencing intense emotions and felt as if they were on a rollercoaster. To work through her grief, Kristen had started to make a book about her pregnancy and the baby, and was spending time with her sister and a friend, talking about the baby and her feelings. Suresh was building a special cubby house in honour of their son.

Accessing therapy or support groups and tapping into online resources including forums can be helpful.

Miscarriage, stillbirth and infertility involve loss and grief, and potentially trauma. Anxiety and depression can result, and seeking support is vital.

Infertility is defined as the inability to conceive after one year of trying, or for women over 35 years, after six months, or the inability to carry a pregnancy to term. The number of women and couples experiencing infertility issues is growing worldwide and is reported to affect 10 to 15 per cent of women of reproductive age. It may be due to causes related to the woman or the man, or may be unexplained.[16]

For those of us who experience infertility and possibly seek reproductive assistance, there are major challenges involved. Managing uncertainty about fertility and coping with the assisted reproduction process can be very stressful for the woman and her partner, and can impact mental health and wellbeing, particularly in relation to stress, anxiety and disturbed mood. As a result, quality of life can be reduced.[17]

Infertility impacts all aspects of life, so a holistic approach is vital. The woman's sense of identity may be impacted and they may feel a sense of guilt, shame, isolation or anger. And cultural or religious beliefs may impact the experience of infertility and be a barrier to seeking help. Reproductive clinics often offer counselling, and therapists can offer support and target concerns such as stress, anxiety, loss and grief and low mood as well as social, sexual or relationship concerns. Engaging in meaningful activities and individual therapy, along with couple counselling, may also be helpful.

A holistic approach is vital: Infertility can impact many aspects of a woman's life. Therapy and support can help with related stress, anxiety, loss and grief and low mood as well as relationship concerns.

Endometriosis is a chronic inflammatory disease, in which cells that are similar to the lining of the uterus grow outside of the uterus and result in pain (including painful periods and painful sex), and possibly infertility issues. The cells can go to the pelvis or abdomen, or even the sciatic nerve (in which pain goes down into the legs).

Endometriosis can be related to anhedonia, or loss of enjoyment in activities that we usually enjoy, as well as anxiety and depression.[18] Seeing a doctor who understands the impacts of endometriosis is important, and treatment may be surgical or hormonal. Pain management (see Chapter 11) and talking therapies play an important role.

Perimenopause and menopause

Menopause refers to the end of the monthly menstrual cycles, whereas perimenopause refers to the time from when the cycle starts changing until twelve months after the final menstrual period. The perimenopause often lasts four to six years but can last up to ten years. During this time oestrogen levels become depleted, and progesterone and testosterone levels also fall. Trans women who lower or stop oestrogen treatment as they age can also experience menopausal symptoms.

Most women begin menopause in their late 40s or early 50s, but there is great variation in timing. The transition into menopause involves major hormonal changes and although some women do not experience symptoms, many do. These include physical as well as psychological and social symptoms. It can be a time of reassessing identity as a result of the changes related to this phase, and our sense of self-worth may be affected.

Symptoms of perimenopause can include physical symptoms such as irregular and variably heavy periods, hot flushes and night sweats, sleep problems, low libido and painful intercourse. Mood swings, anxiety (especially panic episodes) and depression symptoms, irritability or anger, brain fog and cognitive concerns (decline in memory and attention) may also occur.

Menopausal symptoms are similar and can include headaches, night sweats and hot flushes, hair growth or loss, a redistribution of weight to the abdominal area and reduced muscle mass. Vaginal dryness and urinary symptoms may occur. Postmenopausal women may notice that some symptoms continue and others become less noticeable.[19] Coping with the bodily changes can be very challenging.

Perimenopause and menopause involve a great deal of hormonal and life changes, and can involve a number of physical and psychological symptoms.

Depression during perimenopause occurs more often than during the reproductive phase of life. As mentioned earlier, hormones (particularly oestrogen) interact with our brain cells and functioning, and this can impact mood. We may experience depression for the first time, but having a history of depression increases our risk at this time, and women who have had sensitivity at previous times of hormonal change are more at risk. Related sleep disturbances also impact mood.

Apart from low mood and loss of enjoyment in activities that usually provide pleasure, symptoms of depression can include poor sleep, fatigue and irritability. Anxiety is also common. These symptoms can impact daily functioning and relationships at home and at work.[20] We can reflect on these impacts through the story of Carly:

> Carly turned 50 years of age and her partner John suggested a party to celebrate the milestone. Carly could not think of anything worse. She was feeling tired due to her sleep being disrupted by night sweats. She felt more anxious than usual, and wasn't enjoying work. In fact, her colleagues were annoying her a lot, and she preferred to do most of her work from home. John was supportive, but affection and sexual relations seemed to have dwindled. Carly found herself becoming more depressed as time went on.

So what do we do to help Carly, who is struggling with the physical and psychological symptoms associated with menopause? Let's explore this now.

Accessing good quality information about perimenopause and its effects, such as from the Australasian Menopause Society, is important (see 'Resources' on p. 333). There is also an assessment tool available specifically related to depression and perimenopause (see 'Resources' on p. 333). It determines severity of depression and indicates if treatment is needed (generally for moderate or severe depression). Medical assessment and advice is important, and again, perhaps seek out a doctor with a specific interest in women's health.

It can be helpful to have a 'wellbeing plan' at this time. It might look like this:

» Move (e.g. walk each day).

» Connect (with others, with the community).

» Learn (keep reading!).

» Notice (be more mindful).

» Give (to others, the environment, the community).[21]

Perhaps write this list down and put it on your phone or fridge as a reminder!

In relation to the treatment of depression associated with menopause, there is limited research. However, eating healthily, moderating alcohol intake and having regular exercise is known to be important for physical and mental health at this time. Seeing a therapist can also help you navigate this transition, and strategies from Cognitive Behaviour Therapy will be useful (see Chapter 6).

Managing depression during perimenopause: Focus on a healthy lifestyle, having a wellbeing plan, and possibly seeing a therapist. Hormonal therapy or antidepressant medication may have a role.

In terms of medication, hormonal therapy may be suggested during perimenopause or after menopause. In the past there was controversy about the safety of menopausal hormone therapy after a large study was published citing risk. As a result, many women did not seek assistance, endured symptoms and also missed out on many of the preventive benefits of this therapy (on bone, heart and brain health). However, extensive ongoing reviews of this study led to newer hormonal therapies becoming widely accepted as a helpful option for many women.[22]

Menopausal hormone therapy has been shown to assist with perimenopausal or menopausal mood and cognitive issues as well as the physical symptoms, and may be offered if there are no absolute contraindications (mainly previous or current hormone-dependent cancers). It is, of course, important to weigh up individual benefits versus any risks.[23] There is a range of medications to consider as menopausal hormone therapy, including some which are body identical hormones and available on prescription in some countries. There is also medication available to help with hot flushes, and testosterone may be considered to assist with reduced sexual desire.

Antidepressants may be recommended by your doctor to provide assistance with depression or anxiety, especially when symptoms are severe.[24] It is worth talking with a doctor to understand more about these options (including newer agents that are available).

> Carly did decide to talk to her doctor and they did a physical check and talked about strategies that might help, including lifestyle measures and menopausal hormone therapy. There were no contraindications to the therapy, so Carly decided to try it.
>
> Carly and the doctor were concerned about the depressed mood, and met over a number of appointments to talk more. Carly found it good to be listened to as she reviewed life at home and at work. The menopausal hormonal therapy relieved a lot of the physical symptoms, and the depression started to improve, too.

Let's summarize

We have reviewed the menstrual cycle, hormones and mood in this chapter. Their relationship across the life cycle and the various transitions have been explored. We have not been able to address all of the issues affecting women, but we have made a start.

In particular we talked about premenstrual syndromes and their impact on mood, and looked into the link between the various hormones and premenstrual dysphoria. A range of therapies, from complementary and lifestyle measures, to hormonal and antidepressant medications, may be used to relieve symptoms.

Anxiety and depression are common in the perinatal period, and it is vital to address any contributing factors with the woman and potentially her partner. Support from family is important and seeing a therapist can assist. Addressing sleep is vital, and medication may be needed.

Post-partum psychosis is less common and is considered a medical emergency. Urgent assistance is needed.

Miscarriage, stillbirth and infertility are common experiences and are very distressing. The distress may be related to loss and grief, and trauma. Stress, anxiety or depression can occur, and it is important that a holistic approach is taken.

Perimenopause and menopause trigger a wide range of physical and psychological symptoms. Depression can be a significant issue, and it is thought that the fall in oestrogen plays a significant role. Symptoms can be very troublesome and impact functioning and mood. We looked at the various treatments and discussion focused on menopausal hormone therapy, and the role of antidepressant medications.

Here is a summary of the keys from this chapter:

» Help is available to relieve premenstrual symptoms, including working on sleep and using exercise.

» Drop the idea of being a perfect mother.

» Infertility can impact many aspects of a woman's life, so a holistic approach is vital.

» To manage depression during perimenopause, focus on a healthy lifestyle, having a wellbeing plan, and possibly seeing a therapist. Hormonal therapy or antidepressant medication may have a role.

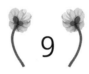

Dealing with relationships and parenting

We have talked about our need for connection with others. We all need a sense of belonging and love as part of our relationships. Let's focus in this chapter on partner relationships, which can bring happiness and be a buffer against challenging events in life.

Our mental health and wellbeing are impacted positively by relationships, but when there are significant issues in the relationship, there can be negative impacts. Equally, when mental health issues such as anxiety, depression or trauma are present, there can be additional stress on relationships.

When a committed relationship ends, there can be significant loss and grief. Divorce and related issues, such as disputes over property and custody of children, can be traumatic and cause great distress.

This chapter will have a focus on prevention, as it is about having a fulfilling partner relationship and preventing relationship problems from arising. We will also consider what can disrupt relationships and how to address the related issues.

Later in the chapter we are going to look at parenting stress, as this influences our relationships. Note that many of the principles covered in this chapter apply equally to heterosexual and same-sex relationships and can be applied to other relationships in life, too. The aim is for relationships to flourish!

Ways to maintain a healthy partner relationship

There are many myths in the community about relationships, created through generations of fairy tales and romantic movies. There may be ideas about finding or being the 'perfect' partner, or that love means an easy path. It is also a myth that each person can be 'everything' to their partner, whereas this is not humanly possible!

Rather than aiming for a fairy tale relationship, the aim is to foster a more secure and healthy relationship. The start of a relationship is often a magical time, during which each person sees the best in their partner and is generous and giving. As time goes on, the relationship becomes more real, and individual flaws become more apparent. There can be disagreements and conflict. Maintaining the relationship becomes very important and this takes effort.

Positive interactions are important: Aim for more positive interactions in relationships, rather than negative ones. To maintain a relationship, we need a good number of positive interactions to compensate for the negative ones.

There are various strategies to help partner relationships over time and to prevent issues from arising, and we are going to go through them now. The strategies relate to connection, communication, caring and compassion, conflict management, creativity and contribution and commitment.

Connection

Humans become 'attached' to other humans, that is, they become linked emotionally and physically. Connection is created through small acts, such as understanding words or a gentle touch, and spending time together. Here are some useful ways to aid connection:

» Be mindful of each other's values, and consider, 'What sort of personal qualities do I want to bring into my relationship?'

» Use empathy and see the world from your partner's point of view. Listen with the aim of understanding.

» Work on letting go of unhelpful stories about the other person or the relationship (such as 'They always let me down').

» Be mindful of your partner generally.

» Connect when you leave your partner (say goodbye), and connect as soon as you come back together (make eye contact and ask how their day was).

» Use 'rituals' to aid connection, such as a regular date night.

Understanding our partner's emotional language(s) can also help a relationship. Author Gary Chapman talks about 'five love languages', suggesting that individuals express their love for their partner in different ways. These are words of affirmation, quality time, receiving gifts, acts of service, and physical touch.[1] It is not often both people in a couple have the same love language, and subsequently they may feel their needs are not being met. It is helpful to spend time working out our own and our partner's language(s) and make efforts to develop and use these languages more.

In addition, therapists John and Julie Gottman speak about the importance of making efforts to 'turn towards' a partner. This means giving a positive response when our partner reaches out for our attention. They may say 'Watch a movie with me' or ask for a hug, and responding to a bid for attention helps our partner feel appreciated and connected. It is important to talk about this together and explore ways to 'turn towards' each other. With couples close to breaking up, bids for attention are often ignored.[2]

In relationships we all make bids for attention and efforts to turn towards our partner. Our partner noticing and responding to these, and vice versa, is important.

Intimacy with a partner involves deep connection. It is about knowing the other person emotionally (their feelings), psychologically (what is on their mind), and physically (touching, sex). Foster connection through validating them with words, gestures (e.g. helping out, giving a gift), and touch (e.g. hugging, kissing, massage).

Communication

Effective communication is essential in relationships. Couples who present for counselling often say communication has failed. What they are saying is that there are issues such as not listening or not being heard, a lack of empathy or dismissing a partner's concerns rather than validating them. It might also refer to not asking regularly about the other person's wellbeing or life, or not letting the partner know they are cared about.

Sometimes we presume that our partner can 'mind read' our needs without us actually talking about them, or we have expectations that they 'should' know about an event or issues. We might avoid communicating about difficult topics, or not be able to express our needs assertively (see p. 183) or respectfully. Passive-aggressive patterns of communicating, such as sarcasm or shutting down, or verbally abusive communication may also arise.

To help communication with a partner, be aware of thinking traps (see p. 101) and avoid ones such as generalizing (e.g. 'You have never understood me'). Instead, focus on understanding your own and your partner's emotions and expressing your emotions. Drop defensiveness and be assertive rather than angry wherever possible, and remember to 'ask nicely' when communicating! We teach children to do this, but sometimes we forget as adults.

Work on communication skills: Avoid criticism, defensiveness, contempt, stonewalling (shutting out the other person). Listen and be calm. Be assertive when needed.

Caring and compassion

Any relationship requires caring and kindness and being a good friend to the other person. When each person is appreciated, they are more likely to be kind to the other. To increase your appreciation, notice three things that you like about our partner, contemplate what your partner adds to your life, reflect on your partner's strengths and say 'thank you' more often.

Caring and compassion require empathy and acknowledging that our partner is sometimes in pain. It is important to look at situations from our partner's perspective and ask, 'Why does this matter to them?'[3] And don't forget self-compassion as well (see p. 49).

Compromise

Each person in a couple needs to tolerate the faults of their partner and be able to compromise or make concessions and find the middle ground. Compromise involves being able to consider the other person's position, accepting the other person's influence and finding some common ground. It also involves accepting the other person's influence to encourage respect and a strong friendship.

When compromise is needed, aim to soften discussion and be calm and respectful. It can help to reflect on a problem separately and then come together to consider what the common feelings and goals are, how the issue can be understood, what can be agreed upon and how the goals can be achieved.

Another useful tool when there is a hard situation to resolve and compromise is necessary comes from Acceptance and Commitment Therapy. Called the LOVE formula, it suggests:

» Letting go of resentment, blaming, judging, criticizing and being demanding

» Opening up to the painful feelings related to the relationship, and to your partner's feelings, acknowledging feelings are important

» Valuing by caring, contributing and connection; connecting with values can assist by helping you focus on what is important to you and not sweating the small things

» Engaging or being psychologically present and able to focus on your partner.[4]

Conflict management

Couples who go to counselling also report problems with conflict in the relationship. This might relate to time spent together and apart, money, health, and gender differences (in heterosexual relationships). The most common causes of conflict are finances, housework, the first child, in-laws and sex.

It has been suggested that in heterosexual relationships, discontent for women often stems from the perception that their partner does not listen when they make an effort to communicate or is unable to meet their emotional needs. Men, on the other hand, may focus on what to do to fix the problem; this might be appropriate, but we may want to first focus on how they feel about the problem.[5]

Interestingly, research indicates that many partner arguments cannot be fully 'resolved'. This is because there may be different views based on previous life experiences (e.g. the type of school a child should go to, or where to invest money). Acceptance of this is important, as is working on a compromise together.

We often head to therapy when there is a lot of conflict. We can improve how we manage conflict, and also accept that not all arguments can be resolved and compromise may be the answer.

Here are some helpful keys to deal with conflict in relationships:

» Be aware of thinking traps which may come into play as conflict escalates. Watch out for unrealistic expectations of the other person.

» Understand that we have the most control over our behaviours rather than our thoughts or feelings. Focus on helpful behaviours, such as listening, and reduce unhelpful ones, such as criticizing.

» When conflict is escalating, take time out from the discussion. Couples need to talk about this together ahead of time, as sometimes in arguments one person will move away and the other person will 'chase' them. Consider how each person feels in this instance (possibly anxious or abandoned) and work out a plan to allow each to have some time out if need be.

» When there are difficult emotions, such as anxiety or hurt, individuals need to be able to soothe themselves, and then each other. We need to let our partner know that we are feeling overwhelmed and need some time out, then do something to feel calmer, such as exercise or meditation. Once both are calm, we are then able to soothe each other.

» Let go of the need to have the last word. This means that we allow ourselves to be vulnerable and open to some painful feelings.

» Be aware of the stories we have developed which feed conflict. One might be the 'It is not safe to trust' story, in which we are hyper-alert for signs of betrayal because of past experiences; and another is the 'housework' story, about who is contributing more or less. These stories can lead to repetitive or 'pet' arguments, and they need to be acknowledged and worked through with understanding.[6]

In addition, at times we need to take responsibility for conflict. It can help to ask ourselves questions like, 'What did I say or do to worsen things? Can I admit some role in creating the conflict? What are some more helpful actions?' Couples often argue about topics associated with control and power. One or each person might be determined to have their own way, but if we expect everyone else to see things the way we do, we are more likely to try to exert power and control over others. This often leads to more and more conflict, and a negative effect on the relationship over time. More flexibility is needed.

There has been a lot written about the need for 'fair fighting'. Too often, individuals use 'dirty fighting' tactics rather than 'fair fighting'. Dirty fighting refers to tactics used to win an argument or inflict pain. Author Russ Harris highlights issues with 'dirty fighting', including:

» going off-topic and unleashing something the person did wrong in the past

» ganging up by getting a third party involved in the argument

» being mean and focusing on something we know will upset the other person

» twisting the other person's words, taking them out of context or exaggerating them

» throwing objects or slamming doors (we will look at domestic violence in a moment).[7]

Part of managing these tactics is having some rules about 'fair fighting'. These rules can help us deal with conflict more effectively and save relationships from breaking down. Asking ourselves why we feel upset, discussing one issue at a time and staying with the topic, and not use degrading language can help. Expressing feelings in words and taking responsibility for them, for example, 'I feel angry and hurt', is important. We need to avoid stonewalling or shutting the other person out, yelling and any physical conflict. The aim is to take time out if need be and to come to a compromise if possible.

Adopt 'fair fighting' rules: They help to resolve conflict by preventing arguments from escalating. We need to stay on topic and not bring in the past. Plus, no ganging up, being mean or twisting words.

The Gottmans also stress the importance of making 'repair attempts' in relationships. These involve words or actions aimed at repairing the relationship after conflict. Practice is often needed to recognize attempts at repair. Focusing on the words being used can help, for example, sentences beginning with 'I feel …' or 'I appreciate …' might be a repair attempt, or statements such as, 'I need to calm down', 'Can we take a rest?' or 'Sorry'.

Conflict can also be about resentment. As discussed in Chapter 7, resentment can build up over time and it can eat away at positive feelings. Examples of issues which might cause resentment include one person perceiving that they are left to do all the housework or child-rearing, or another person believing that they sacrificed their career for the other person. Forgiveness can offer relief from resentment. It means pardoning the person and letting go of resentments. It is not easy, but it is powerful. Remember that forgiveness does not involve forgetting or excusing, but it does involve LOVE: Letting go, Opening up, Valuing and Engaging.

Creativity

Creativity refers to seeing the world in a different way and developing new ideas. We can apply creativity to relationships and help them flourish! We can be creative with problem-solving, and think laterally when coming up with possible solutions. Creativity can be also used to instil some fun and flexibility into relationships, and to revive intimacy. It can be applied to appreciating each other and finding new ways to express this and applying the 'five love languages'.

A good starting point involves creating shared meaning in

relationships. This might involve revisiting values and exploring how things are done in the relationship, such as how birthdays are celebrated. Rituals and celebrations can be important; for example, romance can be woven into rituals to foster intimacy, such as a regular 'date night'. We can also look at how each person is supporting the other and their dreams, and any spiritual dimensions to the relationship can be explored, too.

Let's hear the story of a couple who saw a therapist for couple counselling, and found some creative ways to get their relationship back on track:

Amanda and Lou, a professional couple in their mid-thirties with two young children, were finding that they were arguing more and more and not spending much quality time together. They felt distant from each other. They explored their relationship and shared values with a therapist and talked about their shared goals. The therapist suggested they reconnect with each other by finding more time to be together. They were asked to think about this creatively. Amanda and Lou decided to have regular 'date nights' out and at home. They organized babysitting each fortnight and they also spent time together each weekend planning changes to their garden, and working on it together. Gradually they felt more connected and more content in their relationship.

Tap into creativity: Think about some ways to be more creative in your relationship, such as doing some new things together. Jot down ideas in your journal.

Contribution and commitment

Healthy relationships require both contribution and commitment by partners. Here are some ways to build contribution and commitment:

» Individually, consider the level of commitment to the relationship. Use a scale of 0 to 10, where 0 is no commitment and 10 is the most committed you could be. Is some work needed here?

» Consider the different roles in the relationship, as these will influence the contributions made. Discuss current roles and possibilities for the future.

» Be mindful of unhelpful thinking about expectations of each other, and watch out for any underlying beliefs such as 'being taken for granted', which may push your thinking around.

» Work through life goals together; with specific areas such as finances, discuss concerns and work on managing any issues together.

» Connect with each other and learn the best ways to soothe each other when each is stressed.[8]

Commitment may involve going to couple counselling for a while or intermittently.

Patterns of attachment

Earlier we mentioned attachments, which refers to long-lasting emotional bonds with people we actively want to be close to. There is a theory called 'attachment theory', which talks about our early attachments with parents or caregivers, suggesting that these shape our expectations and behaviours in later relationships.

Research has shown that when parents or caregivers are responsive to their infant's needs, this provides a 'safe base' for the infant to feel secure enough to then explore their world. Developing a secure attachment helps us learn to manage our emotions and helps us in later partner relationships.

Several main patterns or styles of attachment have been identified:

» **Secure style:** The infant learnt that the parent was a safe base and responded to their needs. If an adult has a secure attachment style in childhood, they feel okay with displaying interest and affection, as well as with being alone and independent. They can cope with rejection but report being happiest in relationships. They tend to choose partners well, because they are not interested in being treated badly by others.

» **Insecure avoidant style:** The infant experienced a lack of intimacy with the parent or caregiver. The infant learnt that the parent did not respond to their emotions, especially when they were needy or angry, so they learnt to repress their feelings and become independent. Adults with avoidant attachment are often uncomfortable with intimacy. They may avoid commitment or avoid too much contact with their partners.

» **Insecure ambivalent (or anxious) style:** The infant with this style learnt that even if the parent was physically present, they would sometimes but not necessarily always soothe them. As result they tend to 'overactivate' their attachment system and become clingy. Adults with an anxious attachment style have difficulty being single compared with the other styles and, as a result, are more likely to have unhealthy relationships.

» **Disorganized or chaotic style:** These infants often experienced physical or sexual abuse, and the parent might have had severe mental health or substance-related issues. The infant learnt to be fearful of the parent, as the parent also represented danger. They displayed a chaotic mix of behaviours (moving towards the parent, then away).[9]

It is said that psychological issues occur and interpersonal relationships break down when an individual's need for attachment is not being met. This can occur both when we cannot effectively communicate our needs and when our partner is not able to respond adequately to our needs.

Awareness can help us understand behaviours, be less distressed by them, and work on changing them. When getting to know potential partners we can also be aware of their level of security.

The attachment model can help us understand how we respond in relationships. Here are a few examples of how attachment style can influence our responses, and what me may need to work on:

» If we have an avoidant attachment style we often partner with those with an anxious style. You need to foster your ability to be intimate emotionally with a partner and not pull away, and to allow mutual support.

» If we have an anxious attachment style, we need plenty of reassurance from our partners, and trust issues may occur. If we partner with someone with an avoidant style, there will be challenges. However, for those of us with an anxious style, learning to communicate our needs and choosing secure partners will result in more fulfilling relationships.

>> Adults with the chaotic style of attachment tend to have chaotic relationships, with conflict and many crises.

It is important to remember that change is always possible, thanks to neuroplasticity, and we can work on developing a more secure attachment style over time. This will aid our relationships.

Work on attachment: We can work on having a more secure style of attachment over time. Learning how to clearly communicate our feelings and needs is part of the process.

Fostering a healthy sexual relationship

When we think about a healthy relationship, we tend to think the sexual side has to be good. This part of a relationship is critical to the relationship's health. Research has shown that it is actually the affection and emotional intimacy that accompanies sex that is most important.[10]

Everyday kissing, hugging and touch are key to a relationship. But for various reasons, some people struggle to show affection and sometimes expectations may need to be reduced. They may need to practise affection to learn to be more comfortable with it.

It is important to have affection in a relationship, including everyday affection and during sex. Partners who feel loved and cared for have an improved sexual relationship.

Sex creates connection between partners because they feel more attached. Sexual disconnection, on the other hand, is a common cause of dissatisfaction and distress in relationships and is often talked about in couples therapy. There may be dissatisfaction about differing sex drives and frequency of sex, or about specific sexual issues. Most sexual health issues benefit from attention to the relationship generally, as well as to specific sexual issues.

Nurture partner relationships: Especially the sense of connection and intimacy (e.g. spending more time together talking, adding more light touch or massage into the relationship).

Individuals vary in sex drive, and we also need to take into account physical and mental health issues, medications and stage in life. For example, going through a busy stage in life with young children or overworking may impact sex drive. It can help to have a good look at lifestyles, stress levels and priorities and consider adjusting them if need be.

Nowadays pornography is having an impact on sexual relationships, with some partners being less interested in sex with a partner because of their addiction to pornography and the 'high' that it provides. A partner may also have unrealistic expectations of what sexual acts a partner may be comfortable in engaging with due to the pornography.

Normal sexual responding may also be disrupted. The causes of sexual dysfunction will vary, but will be related to physical or psychological functioning, or the relationship. There will be an overlap between physical, psychological and relationship factors.

Perhaps start with a check-up to explore any physical factors that may be contributing, such as pain or vaginal atrophy around menopause. It is important to look at general health, too, such as exercise, alcohol use and reducing stress. A doctor can assist with referrals to a counsellor or sex therapist and advise on whether medication might be helpful (e.g. testosterone might be considered around menopause).

Mental health disorders such as anxiety and depression may be related to issues with sexual functioning, as can the medication used in treatment. Past trauma can also have a significant impact. (Take some time to read about these issues if relevant in Chapters 4, 6 and 10.)

Also consider whether 'performance anxiety' is having an impact. Sex is about intimacy and enjoyment, rather than performance and achieving orgasm, so lessen the need to self-monitor, and stop self-criticism. Relax the body and be mindful and focus on all the pleasurable sensations. Hypnotherapy may assist in lessening this form of anxiety.

Things that can disrupt relationships

Life is all about relationships but sometimes things can go wrong within them. We cannot look at all the potential problems that can arise, but we will consider a few. We need to recognize them and deal with them early. This may involve seeking out some help from supports and professionals. We will look at a few important relationship issues, namely infidelity, intimate partner abuse and violence, narcissistic personality, and also separation and divorce.

Infidelity

An **affair** refers to an intense emotional or sexual relationship (sex or inappropriate physical contact) with someone other than our partner.[11] Dealing with infidelity is very difficult for a couple. It is a painful process due to the distress caused and can have a very destructive effect on the relationship.

Social media has led to a new type of affair. What may start out as a flirtation can lead to a significant 'emotional affair' and an addiction to the thrill of online involvement with someone. Emotional affairs are more common than sexual affairs. Research has found that women are more upset about emotional affairs, and men are more concerned about sexual affairs.

An affair is a sexual or emotional relationship with someone other than our partner.

There are several potential causes of infidelity. It may be that monogamy is a struggle for an individual. We know that people who are unfaithful in one relationship are more likely to be unfaithful in their next one, compared to those who have not been unfaithful in the first one. There may be a lack of emotional connection between partners, or possibly emotional dissatisfaction in the relationship. And if aspects of the relationship are triggering low self-worth, this may contribute. There may also be underlying problems stemming from past trauma or sexual addictions.

Healing from an affair involves acknowledging and talking about what has happened. If the affair involved a sexual relationship, having a check for sexually transmitted infections is vital. For the relationship to survive, the affair must end, and we need to recognize that we can only be responsible for our own fidelity. It can help to seek out couples therapy to explore what happened, the associated feelings and any underlying issues in the relationship.

An affair involves a very significant breach of trust. This needs to be rebuilt and this takes time. The partner who has broken the trust must be willing to explore their actions to see what has contributed, and the couple needs to look at the relationship and any problem areas.

Trust must be earned again via actions, including speaking honestly and being reliable. Sometimes amends may need to be made by validating the other person's feelings, expressing remorse, apologizing for the hurt, showing more appreciation for the other person and spending time together. Focus on trusting in small ways first, then gradually larger actions of trust can be taken.

It is important to trust our intuition. Sometimes acceptance is needed, that we may never be certain that the partner will not repeat the behaviours, but that they are committed and making an effort. At times, an individual will see a therapist because they are feeling guilty about the affair. They want to tell the other person to ease their own distress. However, this should not be the main motivation for telling a partner. We need to put our partner's needs ahead of our own in this situation and then make a decision.

Also, the result of an affair may be that a couple decide to have a more open relationship. This involves being committed to the relationship but having sex outside the relationship and being honest about this. Some people can manage this, but many others can't. Those individuals with a more anxious attachment style will struggle with this, and anxiety and jealousy can arise.

Intimate partner abuse or violence

Intimate partner abuse or violence can occur no matter what our age, gender or sexual orientation. One in four Australian women has experienced violence and abuse by a current or former partner, and it is widely reported that violence increased during the COVID-19 pandemic. Women with existing mental health disorders are at greater risk. Femicide is the most extreme form of gender-based violence.[12] This violence is a major public health concern and a violation of human rights.[13]

Some communities, such as Australia's Aboriginal and Torres Strait Islander communities, prefer the term 'family violence'. Family violence refers to violence between family members (e.g. children and parents), as well as intimate partners.

The abuse or violence results in, or is likely to result in, physical, sexual or psychological harm or suffering to women. Intimate partner abuse and violence is one of the leading causes of disability and death in women of childbearing age.[14]

The related disability may involve painful conditions, hearing loss, kidney and urinary infections, sexually transmitted infections, chronic pelvic pain or irritable bowel syndrome. It may be associated with depression, substance-related issues, suicidality and post-traumatic stress disorder (and complex post-traumatic stress disorder) (see Chapters 6, 7 and 10).[15]

Almost 90 per cent of intimate partner violence is perpetrated by men against women. Physical and sexual violence against women by men is considered to be used as a means to maintain male dominance in families and sustain masculine identity. There may be an ingrained belief that men's needs (including sexual) are to be met by women. This entitlement has been linked to rape, intimate partner violence, sexual abuse of children, sexual harassment and economic abuse.[16]

Intimate partner abuse and violence are used to control and dominate the other person, and this causes fear and potentially physical or psychological harm. It can involve physical or sexual assault, verbal, emotional, psychological or financial abuse, deprivation of liberties, coercion, intentionally causing injury or death to a pet, threats, damage to property or stalking.[17]

Coercive control is a pattern of actions that aim to cause fear and result in control. This may include social control (isolating the woman from friends or family), and technology-facilitated abuse (such as tracking movements or monitoring text messages). Mental health coercion may involve threatening suicide to manipulate the woman. Migrant and refugee women may be manipulated by the perpetrator related to their visa status.[18]

Here are a few important points about intimate partner abuse and violence:

» Intimate partner abuse and violence is dangerous. It can be life-threatening, and safety is the priority.

» It can include physical assault (including strangulation and choking), sexual assault, verbal abuse, emotional abuse, financial abuse, technology-facilitated abuse, social abuse (isolating someone from their supports) or spiritual abuse (stopping someone from practising their religion).

» At the centre of abuse is a controlling behaviour pattern. It may include going through a partner's text messages, emails and social media, controlling money, criticizing continuously, ignoring the person or refusing to talk, or emotional blackmail, for example, 'If you loved me, you would …' In a relationship, threats to hurt, kill or rape can be about control.

» There is often a cycle of violence, that is, there is a tension-building phase with conflict and abuse, followed by a peak of violence (an 'explosion'). A honeymoon phase follows, with remorse and promises of no more violence. There can be denial of the problem during this phase.

» This cycle repeats itself over time, and the abuse tends to increase in severity and frequency over time.

» It is important to have a 'safety plan' in place (what to do, who to contact, where to go) to deal with dangerous situations.

» The most dangerous time for a woman in an abusive relationship is at separation, and many women live in fear of reprisals after leaving.[19]

» When a partner has significant personality issues, such as narcissistic personality traits or disorder (see the next section), they may be more likely to perpetrate abusive behaviours.

Emergency help: If there is an emergency in relation to intimate partner violence we need to phone the emergency services number in our location.

Some people find it hard to understand why we struggle to leave abusive relationships. However, there are many possible reasons. Abuse and violence can build gradually, and there are cycles during which the perpetrator is apologetic. Over time, control increases and leaves us feeling trapped (often for good reasons, such as threats) and self-worth and sense of identity is eroded. Mental health and wellbeing may be significantly impacted, contributing to the challenge to leave. The woman may be protecting children and be aware of the risks attached to leaving.

Women need to be alert to the nature of abuse and seek help. (Equally, if the woman is abusing another person, responsibility needs to be taken and help sought.) Most countries will have government websites and services (such as national phone hotlines) addressing intimate partner abuse and violence. Seeing a doctor might be a first step. They can do a risk assessment and advise on available supports. Some therapists specialize in this area or there may be group programs available. Support agencies may also be able to assist a person leaving an abusive relationship with shelter, financial and emotional support.

Narcissistic personality disorder

We may all potentially have some narcissistic personality traits, but a personality disorder represents an enduring pattern of experience and behaviour that impacts interpersonal relationships and other areas of functioning.[20] Narcissistic personality disorder is one type of personality disorder and may be due to genetics or life experiences. It doesn't refer to someone who is simply confident, assertive or has high self-belief.

Those with narcissistic personality disorders often have an exaggerated sense of their own importance and superiority, and a strong sense of entitlement and need for attention. They lack empathy and tend to exploit others. They can be arrogant and jealous of others. The narcissistic tendencies can be overt (grandiose attitudes, self-assured, dominant) or covert (anxious, overly sensitive, defensive, depressive and withdrawn).[21]

Underneath it all, the person with a narcissistic personality disorder is highly insecure with a fragile sense of self-worth and often a strong sense of shame. This is why controlling or abusing a partner serves to help the person feel more powerful. Some behaviours are very characteristic of narcissistic abuse. These include:

» blaming the partner

» isolating them from loved ones

» baiting and starting arguments

» stonewalling, or withdrawing completely for hours or days

» gaslighting, which refers to creating distrust of our perceptions about reality or our mental wellbeing. Examples of gaslighting might be 'I didn't say that', 'It didn't happen,' '[The threat] was a joke' or 'I'm worried you are going crazy'.

The nature of narcissism, particularly lack of empathy, and its behaviours are very challenging for a partner.

There is often a cycle in the relationship, namely idealizing the partner, then devaluing them and finally discarding them. Early on the narcissistic person may be charming and give extravagant displays of affection and see their partner as perfect, but over time they will criticize their partner, manipulate and blame them. The final stage involves discarding the partner, sometimes abruptly, but they often continue to say and do hurtful things.[22]

Treatment of narcissistic personality disorder involves treatment of related problems such as anxiety or depression. The person needs to develop an awareness that their personality is impacting relationships and want to actively participate in therapy. This is often a challenge and commitment to therapy may not occur. Therapy involves working on current behaviours and attitudes, and managing emotions. It can also involve looking at early life experiences and this tends to be a longer-term approach via psychodynamic or schema-focused psychotherapy. Successful treatment is not assured.

What can you do when in a relationship with a person with a narcissistic personality disorder?

» Realize there is a problem.

» Learn about narcissism and all the related behaviours.

» Reflect on your own responses to the behaviours (such as buying into the blame).

» Prioritize your mental health and wellbeing.

» Set firm boundaries where possible (see Chapter 7).

» Stay connected with family and friends wherever possible.

» Know that you cannot rescue or heal them — they need to do that.

» Consider options for the relationship (counselling, continuing versus ending).

» Seek professional advice and support for yourself.

» If separating, aim to make any discussions or responses brief and avoid getting drawn into conflict.

» And again, keep safe.

Dealing with narcissism: You need to learn about it, and consider whether the relationship is actually what you have been thinking it is and whether it is functional. You can make decisions about the future from there.

Separation and divorce

Separation and divorce are now common. There are some signs that a long-term relationship will eventually end, including a readiness for conflict, failed attempts to mend a relationship after conflict, in combination with criticism, defensiveness, contempt and shutting down. One or both partners may rewrite or change the relationship stories about the past (such as 'We should never have gotten together, we weren't suited'), or the couple is leading parallel lives or feel lonely.

There can be a rollercoaster of emotions around separation, from sadness to anger, fear, overwhelm, guilt or relief. We are unlikely to function as well, with home and work activities affected by sleep issues and difficulty concentrating. With separation and divorce, there can be multiple losses, including family, friends, home and home routines, contact with children, dreams for the future and finances. Our attachments (to others) are disrupted when a relationship ends and significant distress, grief, anxiety or depression can occur.

Recent research has shown that there are some protective factors for our physical and mental health after divorce, related to income, previous divorces and new partner status. However, higher levels of divorce conflict are a risk factor for mental health, highlighting the importance of supporting women who experience higher levels of conflict around divorce.[23]

Adapting to the losses and working through the grief of divorce takes time and it can be a bumpy ride (see Chapter 6). The practical issues, such as financial settlements and child custody issues, may also take significant time. It can be helpful to seek support from a doctor or therapist and, at times, crisis intervention may be necessary, such as if attending to any signs of depression or anxiety and suicide risk. (Refer to Chapters 6 and 7 for more information on loss and grief, depression and managing suicidal thoughts).

Separation and divorce often trigger loss and grief, and our attachments are disrupted.

Here are some general strategies for managing the range of emotions related to separation and divorce and supporting our mental health and wellbeing:

» Take a day at a time, and recognize that recovery takes time.

» Look after yourself and practise self-care (keep eating, exercising and sleeping).

» As much as possible, continue with normal activities and routines, such as seeing friends.

» Prioritize the most important tasks to attend to, such as being there for children.

» Keep talking to supportive family or friends about how things are.

» Express emotions through helpful means, such as writing in your journal, and use self-soothing and distraction activities (see Chapter 7).

» Avoid unhelpful coping strategies such as using alcohol or substances, or any risk-taking activities.

» Find a doctor or therapist to talk to (relationship services may be a good start).

> » Work through loss and grief (see Chapter 6).

> » Work towards acceptance of the separation or divorce, and acknowledge a new path in life and the need to rebuild.

> » Set clear boundaries with former partners in relation to socializing, doing things for them and physical relationship (see Chapter 6).

> » Look after your finances and seek financial counselling if needed.

> » Also seek out advice and support from a lawyer when needed. Knowing your legal rights is vital, and having assistance with formal arrangements such as parenting may be necessary.

> » Consider what you want your new life to look like and work towards that.[24,25]

Recovery takes time: Whether we instigate separation and divorce, or our partner does, the grieving process takes time. Adaption and recovery involves working through emotion, losses and practical challenges. And it involves creating a new life.

Parenting stress

This section is not about parenting skills, as there are many books available on this. Overall, being a parent is associated with psychological wellbeing and life satisfaction, but for some women, mental health and wellbeing may suffer.[26]

We go through stages as a parent, from preparing for the arrival of the baby to our children leaving home, to being there when they need us as adults. Each stage can bring particular stresses, some of which are very normal. We may worry that our infant is meeting their milestones in relation to development, or that they are okay at day care, or whether our child has friends. Some stresses, however, cause significant distress, and relationships may be positively or negatively impacted.

We often have amazing expectations of becoming a parent. Maybe we want to be a great mother, or maybe we want our child to above all else be 'happy and healthy'. Sometimes these expectations are met and sometimes they are not. There can be various reasons for this, some within our control and many outside of our control. There are often competing demands, too, such as managing work and being a parent, or caring for elderly parents at the same time.

Being a parent can be associated with happiness, joy and wellbeing, and there can be other emotions such as guilt or anger, and at times anxiety or depression can result (see Chapter 4 and 6). Our own issues (such as trauma) from childhood and our parenting may be triggered. Or we may be a sole parent or co-parent and facing particular challenges, and housing or financial issues may also contribute to the stress.

We often have expectations (or beliefs) about parenthood or ourselves as a parent. Society gives us many messages about what being a mother should be. One is that we are ideally a 'natural mother', whether this means being able to breastfeed a baby, intuitively knowing what to do to settle a baby, or having a well-behaved child. Another is being the 'perfect mother'. Feelings of guilt or shame can result. Remember that in this instance, reality most often does not measure up to these ideals, as the related expectations are unrealistic (see p. 216).

Myths about women and being a mother, and in recent years images of 'the perfect mother' on social media, have all contributed to these ideas. As a result we might think we should be fully in control of the situation and totally responsible when these things are not happening. Self-criticism can grow and guilt and shame may follow (see Chapter 3). Women are particularly vulnerable to these influences during the postnatal period (see Chapter 8).

The 'perfect mother' does not exist in reality!

Remember that babies and children have different temperaments and needs. Some have special needs, such as children with cerebral palsy or attention deficit hyperactivity disorder, or autistic children. The overall aim is to love the child, keep them safe and help them reach their potential, but this is all dependent on the parent maintaining their own wellbeing as best as they can (see Chapter 7).

The COVID-19 pandemic has added additional layers of stress with many women impacted by changes at hospitals at the time of birthing (often with lack of supports being present), or not being able to go out with babies or small children due to infections in the community. These factors have been shown to have significantly impacted mental health and wellbeing.[27] The effects of the pandemic on work, childcare and schooling have also been significant, contributing to the sense of exhaustion mentioned in Chapter 7.

> Sophia and Daniel were parents to three children. Two were teenagers and there was a younger one, too. Life was busy with work, home and all of the children's activities. Sophia never seemed to have a moment to herself and if she did have a moment, she needed to touch base with her mother, who had some health problems.
>
> Then COVID-19 hit and everyone was working and schooling from home. Sophia had an additional role, being a teacher. And the teenagers were not happy: missing out on their friends, sporting finals and school celebrations. She had no idea how she would cope. She was already exhausted, and something had to give!
>
> In the end Sophia talked to a friend and they empathized with each other. The friend suggested a few strategies like meditation and exercise, and talking with Daniel about lightening the load. Sophia found some useful ideas online and bit by bit she made some changes. She knew that she had to.

Here are some suggestions to manage parenting stress and reduce burnout:

» Recognize your own expectations and consider whether they are realistic.

» Drop comparisons with others.

» Look for new perspectives, especially when having a tough moment ('Is there another way to think about this?') or when being self-critical (see Chapter 3).

» Adopt strategies to reduce stress, such as meditation, exercise or delegating tasks at home (to a partner, other family, or hiring help if possible).

» Remember self-care, such as eating regularly, getting sleep when possible, and some exercise.

» Keep things simple. Focus on what is important and drop things that don't fit with this, especially with a baby or infant.

» Practise mindfulness each day, such as watching a child play or being out in nature with them, and use your senses to enjoy the moment.

» Notice and acknowledge the 'good' moments. Practise gratitude.

» Trust yourself and your intuition.

» Grow your support networks, whether family, friends, community or online and tap into them. Utilize reputable apps for information and support.

» Talk about what is going on and related emotions with trusted people. Express emotions in constructive ways.

» Work on organizing supports for children with special needs.

» Remember that babies, infants, children and teenagers pass through stages and grow! There is often calm after a stormy patch.

» Monitor your mental health and wellbeing.

» Seek professional support as needed. Seeing a doctor is a good start or see a therapist.

Coping with parenting stress: Remember that sometimes we take a few steps forward and then some back. The key is to keep on stepping with small steps!

Let's summarize

Relationships can bring great joy, and also challenges. To maintain healthy partner relationships and therefore assist our mental health and wellbeing, focus on the 'Cs' outlined in the chapter, namely, connection, communication, caring and compassion, compromise and conflict management, creativity, and contribution and commitment. Within each of these areas there are many helpful strategies, such as practising paying attention, communicating effectively and using the LOVE formula. Fostering emotional intimacy and a healthy sexual relationship are important.

We looked at some of the problems that can occur in relationships, including infidelity, intimate partner abuse and violence, living with a partner with narcissistic personality disorder, and separation and divorce. Understanding these issues means we are more aware, and more likely to reach out for support and assistance. Safety is the priority.

The chapter also explored patterns of attachment in relationships, as understanding these can help us be aware of how we, or our partners, are responding in relationships. And thanks to neuroplasticity, we can work on a more secure attachment style over time.

Stress associated with being a parent was discussed, and COVID-19 has added a layer of stress. Parenting can be associated with great satisfaction in life, and at times great stress. We looked at managing our expectations of ourselves and the importance of self-care.

Here is a summary of the keys highlighted in this chapter:

» Positive interactions are important; aim for more positive than negative ones.

» Work on communication skills.

» Adopt 'fair fighting' rules.

» Tap into creativity.

» Work on attachment.

» Nurture partner relationships, especially the sense of connection and intimacy.

» Emergency help: If there is an emergency in relation to intimate partner violence you need to *phone the emergency services number in your location.*

» Dealing with narcissism: Learn about it, and consider whether the relationship is actually what you have been thinking it is and whether it is functional.

» Recovery takes time: Whether you instigate separation and divorce, or your partner does, the grieving process takes time.

» Coping with parenting stress: Remember that sometimes we take a few steps forward and then some back.

The impact of abuse
and trauma

Trauma is probably the most underestimated influence on mental
health. We see the effects of trauma in practice over and over again.
Trauma is defined as the broad psychological and neurobiological
effects of an event, or series of events, which produce experiences of
overwhelming fear, stress, helplessness or horror.[1] Examples of trauma
are accidents, assaults or hearing traumatic news about a loved one.

In this chapter we will look at the causes and the impact of trauma
in our lives. Unfortunately, trauma is a common experience for women,
especially sexual trauma. We have already considered intimate partner

violence in Chapter 9, and in this chapter we will consider childhood sexual abuse and sexual assault, among other causes of trauma.

We will also focus on recovery from trauma. Thanks to neuroplasticity, healing can occur. It may take time, support and work, but there are many approaches that can help. We will explore the principles behind them and some of the strategies they use. It is wonderful when recovery opens the door to flourishing in life.

> Please be aware that reading about trauma can potentially be triggering (or may activate anxiety) for women who have experienced trauma, so please be mindful of this and choose if, when and how, this chapter can be read and processed.

We are first going to look at what we know about trauma.

Possible causes

Traumatic events are often unexpected, negative, pose a threat to safety and may be life-threatening. Any event that involves a threat to life or a serious injury has the potential to be traumatic. This includes experiencing natural disasters (see p. 129), an accident, and physical or sexual assault. Trauma can occur any time in life, from childhood through to old age.

Trauma associated with medical procedures is an example that can impact at any age. And those of us working in health in various capacities have a risk of trauma related to the nature of our work, especially during COVID-19, and also from vicarious trauma that can result from hearing the stories of our client's trauma.

It is particularly important to look at childhood trauma, which may involve a single incident or repeated physical, verbal or sexual abuse, or physical and emotional neglect. Trauma may also occur when a parent abuses alcohol or is diagnosed with a serious mental health issue, or when a parent leaves the family or passes away. Bullying in childhood is also a common cause of trauma.

Trauma in adult life may be related to an accident, a natural disaster or being assaulted. It can also be due to ongoing abuse in a relationship, or result from childhood abuse.

Facts and figures

Let's consider a few of the facts and figures about trauma and women. They are very concerning:

» It is estimated that one in three women worldwide experience either inmate partner violence or non-partner sexual violence in their lifetime.[2]

» It is estimated that one in five women has survived a rape or attempted rape, and one in four girls experience childhood sexual abuse.[3]

» 10 to 12 per cent of women experience post-traumatic stress disorder in their lifetimes (double the rate of men), often the result of trauma at a younger age.[4]

» Trauma is more common in population groups that have a higher incidence of intergenerational trauma, such as refugees or First Nations peoples.[5]

» Women experiencing severe mental health disorders are at a much greater risk of experiencing trauma, such as assault;[6] and almost half of women admitted to an inpatient facility had a history of childhood sexual and physical abuse.[7]

» A study of adverse experiences in childhood found there was a greater risk of suicide, eating disorders or substance-related issues when there had been traumatic events in childhood.[8]

» Early trauma may also impact our physical health and wellbeing, such as painful conditions or stress-related health issues.[9]

Neurobiology and the impact of trauma

We are going to look at how trauma can affect the nervous system. Remember from Chapter 4 that our nervous system is wired to respond to threats. Trauma activates the automatic (or autonomic) part of the nervous system to help us survive, and it is the sympathetic arm that is responsible for our fight or flight response. The parasympathetic arm has dorsal vagal nerves that trigger the freeze response (immobilizing us). Various stress hormones are released and the fight, flight or freeze response jumps into action.

Children and adolescents and survivors of sexual violence most commonly freeze. This means they are more likely to experience dissociation (such as feeling out of our body or the moment), and this can lead to greater risk of post-traumatic stress disorder. Hyper-vigilance (or the mind scanning for threats) may also continue after a freeze response.[10,11]

When we have been affected by trauma, we are also likely to have a greater response to any later stress or threat. This means that a larger amount of stress hormones is released and they cause symptoms like a rapid heart rate, breathlessness and sweating. In a situation where there is trauma, anxiety can become linked to a trigger. For example, after a car accident, seeing a particular type of car might trigger anxiety.

Studies have shown that brain chemicals, such as serotonin, are affected in trauma, and this is thought to be why irritability, anger and depression may occur. There have also been studies on what happens in the brain itself with trauma. Children are particularly at risk because their brain is growing. A child's limbic brain (see p. 46) can be affected, potentially leading to more extreme emotions and a reduced ability to learn.[12]

It is worth talking about memory and trauma, too. We store a whole lot of information through our memories as 'networks', including sensory information about the experience (the sounds, sights, smells), the experiences of our body, our own responses and the meaning or interpretation we give the experience (such as 'I don't have control' or 'Nowhere is safe'). When there is a trauma, memory may be stored in an unprocessed way, which means we haven't integrated the experience and put it away in our long-term memory. It can therefore be readily activated by triggers, which tends to be involuntary, and this can feel as if the memory is happening now. They are sensory, vivid and emotional, and might occur in the day or night.

We are going to now look at the potential immediate (acute) and longer-term responses to trauma.

Acute stress response

As adults, we will respond in the aftermath of a trauma in different ways depending on our past and our personality. The type and extent of the trauma will have an influence. When trauma occurs, we may respond with a great deal of distress, often triggered by uninvited memories of the event, or distressing dreams and flashbacks (reliving the event with images, sounds or smells). This acute stress response, which may last for the first few weeks, might also involve feeling dissociated or unable to experience feelings of happiness. We may make efforts to avoid any reminders of the trauma and be overly vigilant, unable to concentrate, or are more irritable or angry.

Generally, these feelings often resolve on their own, and with the support of family and friends the individual recovers.

In the first days and weeks after a traumatic event, individuals often experience strong emotions, relive the experience or feel separate or dissociated.

Post-traumatic stress disorder

In contrast, post-traumatic stress disorder involves the development of long-lasting anxiety following a traumatic event (more than a month). The rates of this disorder are higher in countries with a lot of conflict, or in military personnel compared with the general population.

Post-traumatic stress disorder involves a number of ongoing difficulties:

» Reliving the traumatic event through unwanted memories and sensations (e.g. sounds, smells), vivid nightmares, flashbacks or intense reactions when reminded of the event.

» Feeling wound up, that is, having trouble sleeping or concentrating, feeling angry or irritable, taking risks, becoming easily startled, or constantly being vigilant or on the lookout for danger.

» Avoiding reminders of the event, such as activities, places, people, thoughts or feelings that bring back memories of the trauma.

» Uncomfortable thoughts and feelings, including feeling afraid, angry, guilty, depressed or numb a lot of the time, losing interest in day-to-day activities, feeling cut off from friends and family.

Post-traumatic stress disorder refers to persistent anxiety following trauma. Re-experiencing through memories and avoidance of related activities are characteristic.

Trauma may cause difficulties relating to other people, such as family members or partners, as well as with work colleagues. And it is also not unusual for people with post-traumatic stress disorder to experience other mental health problems like depression or anxiety, or substance-related issues (used as a way of coping).

Assessment tools are available for trauma, such as the post-traumatic stress disorder checklist. The various treatment approaches for post-traumatic stress disorder will be outlined later in the chapter.

Sexual trauma

Most people who access sexual assault services are women. Sexual assault includes rape, attempted rape, aggravated sexual assault (with a weapon), indecent assault and forced sexual activity. Sexual assault can occur in a partner relationship. Initially the focus is on emergency care and safety, dealing with injuries and gathering forensic information.[13]

Psychological first aid is vital after sexual assault as there has often been a real or perceived threat to life. Many of us will experience an acute stress response with anxiety, vivid recollections, disturbed sleep and disturbed mood. Being validated and listened to at this stage is important. Going into details is not part of first aid (it may be part of collecting evidence) — the emphasis is on feeling safe and supported.

Referral to a sexual assault service for ongoing care can be made. The acute stress response may resolve, or if symptoms persist, post-traumatic stress disorder may be diagnosed. Coping with later legal or court issues can re-traumatize, and many women do not report assaults due to concerns about the system.

Complex trauma

'Complex trauma' or 'complex post-traumatic stress disorder' are fairly recent terms. Complex trauma can occur when multiple traumatic events occur over a period of time, often involving situations from which escape is difficult or impossible. Examples are child abuse or prolonged intimate partner or family violence.

Complex trauma survivors are likely to experience post-traumatic stress disorder and may have mental health issues such as depression or anxiety, problems with dissociative episodes or psychotic symptoms (see Chapter 11). Personality and self-worth can be affected, along with the ability to have stable relationships or to regulate emotions.[14]

In complex trauma, post-traumatic stress disorder symptoms are present, and in addition there can be:

» problems in regulating emotions

» having negative self-beliefs such as feeling defeated or worthless, accompanied by feelings of shame, guilt or failure related to the trauma

» difficulties in sustaining relationships and in feeling close to others.

These symptoms cause significant impairment in personal, family, social, educational, occupational or other important areas of functioning. Self-harm can occur, especially if there is depression.[15,16]

Recovery from trauma

If you have been impacted by trauma, it is important to seek some help and support. Family and friends may assist, and a doctor can assess the issues and offer guidance, support and treatment. A therapist who knows about the treatment of trauma-related issues needs to be located. Help from a psychiatrist may also be needed.

Therapists will generally take a 'trauma-informed approach', meaning they realize the widespread effects of trauma, recognize the symptoms and respond with empathy as much as possible, as well as creating a sense of safety. This way, a high level of trust is established, and this enables you to be able to share your feelings and tackle the issues. An opportunity to develop a sense of control of the process is provided, and using existing strengths to aid recovery is encouraged.

Therapy for trauma generally focuses on various trauma-focused interventions, and on reducing the symptoms related to the trauma. Approaches that lessen anxiety and depression and improve quality of life will be incorporated.

The foundation of treatment

Before we go on to look into specific therapies, let's briefly revisit an earlier discussion about our nervous systems, as this is what treatment is based on.

Parts of the brain	Effect of trauma	Aim of treatment
The brainstem helps us survive when there is stress or threat.	Various stress hormones are released, and the fight, flight or freeze response occurs.	Reduce activity here.
The limbic brain (the amygdala, insula and hippocampus) is responsible for emotions and memory. Trauma is mostly processed in this area.	The amygdala becomes hyper-reactive to any stimuli related to the trauma. Our hippocampus can be dysregulated and we re-experience the trauma. It can be impacted by chronic stress (prolonged effects of trauma), thought to be related to effects of stress hormones.	Reduce activity in the amygdala. Increase activity in the insula (processes body memories). Increase memory processing (including bodily sensations) and storage.

Parts of the brain	Effect of trauma	Aim of treatment
The cortex houses language, timekeeping, imagination and awareness, and is responsible for decision-making and judgment.[17] This area also helps with regulating emotions.	Functions can be disrupted, for example cognition and also timekeeping (getting pulled back into the past).[18] Changes to brain chemicals, particularly in the cortex, play a part in irritability and mood.	Increase activation here.

As a result of our understanding of the brain, the general treatment approach — referred to as the 'bottom-up' or 'top-down' approach — has been developed. It refers to working with the body to change the brain and/or working with the mind to change the brain.[19] Ideally, treatment involves both approaches.

Here are some examples. Bottom-up work might involve grounding or relaxation techniques, yoga, exercises related to awareness of the body and exposure techniques. Top-down work might involve cognitive therapy or aspects of Acceptance Commitment Therapy. Another therapy that is widely used now in trauma is Eye Movement Desensitization and Reprocessing, which works bottom-up and horizontally, meaning it activates both sides of our brain (see later in the chapter). Art Therapy works in a similar way.[20,21]

Bottom-up and top-down approaches: Involves working with the body to change the brain, and working with the mind, too. Ideally, treatment involves both approaches.

An integrated approach

As mentioned at the outset, an integrative treatment approach is often most helpful. It can incorporate the bottom-up and top-down approaches we have just talked about, and take a holistic approach. Individual or group programs may be involved.

In relation to trauma this might include:

» trauma-informed and supportive care

» addressing all aspects of ourselves (physical, emotional, social, spiritual)

» having plenty of information about trauma and its effects

» addressing lifestyle issues (sleep, exercise, alcohol use and more)

» engaging in meaningful activities and work

» maintaining connections with others

» working on connection with the body through sensory awareness and activities such as yoga

» learning coping skills, including stress management, sleep hygiene, relaxation, grounding, mindfulness and interpersonal skills

» learning self-soothing and emotion regulation skills (see Chapter 7)

» focusing on strengths and values

» utilizing the various evidence-based talking therapies (see p. 46)

» working with the meaning attached to the trauma (more on this shortly)

» managing the associated problems, such as anxiety/depression, substance use or anger

» growing self-belief

» considering medication if needed

» knowing about and using supports and resources.

A holistic and integrated approach can be tailored to address the impact of the trauma on all aspects of ourselves.

The integrative approach is applicable to the various types of trauma we have discussed. With complex trauma there will also be emphasis on:

» appropriately investigating any physical symptoms

» learning ways to regulate emotions (see Chapter 7)

» working on more secure attachment patterns (see p. 241)

» in childhood sexual abuse, dealing with related emotions such as shame and recognizing that the person to blame is not ourselves, but the perpetrator

» Exposure Therapy in relation to avoidance or symptoms such as flashbacks

» reducing self-criticism and growing self-belief

» developing interpersonal skills or working on relationship issues.[22]

Working with blame and shame: The perpetrator of abuse and violence is the responsible one. Letting go of self-blame and personal shame is an important part of healing.

Therapies

Let's look now at some of the available specific therapies for working with trauma.

Trauma-focused Cognitive Behaviour Therapy

This is a specific form of Cognitive Behaviour Therapy, but much of what we have already covered in relation to Cognitive Behaviour Therapy in Chapters 4 and 6 still applies. This approach views trauma as a 'prism' through which we view ourselves, others and the world.[23]

Various behavioural techniques are involved, such as providing information, scheduling pleasant activities, self-care, setting goals, using relaxation techniques, problem-solving and assertiveness training. Note that when the freeze response has been a part of the trauma, grounding techniques may be more helpful, as feeling relaxed may be associated with freezing and could actually trigger anxiety.

Exposure techniques (see p. 100) are also used. These techniques help in dealing with the memories of the traumatic experience(s) in a controlled and safe way. Exposure involves gradually recalling and thinking about memories until they no longer create high levels of distress. This may be done with a therapist through talking or writing in the session, or written exercises at home. This therapy particularly focuses on our sense of safety. A therapist may ask us to consider the relevance of safety in our lives and to identify situations in which we feel vulnerable or triggered. We then talk about what it is about those situations (thoughts, images) that is activating, and how we have handled these situations.

Exposure might then involve visiting a range of related places, recognizing that the traumatic event is unlikely to happen again, that we don't have control over everything that happens to us and that we can't control the behaviour of others. Although the possibility of being exposed to trauma still exists, we can take steps to reduce the possibility of harm to ourselves. It also involves looking at any unhelpful thinking patterns, underlying beliefs or meaning related to the trauma. Here are some examples:

» 'I'm worthless' or 'I'm not the same person'.
» '[My family/partner] is not part of the same story.'
» 'The world is not safe.'
» 'It wasn't fair.'

Once we are aware of our thoughts or beliefs, we can work with the therapist on challenging them and gradually reconstruct our view of ourselves, others and the world. Let's hear two stories to illustrate how this might be done:

Paula had a car accident and sustained some physical injuries and felt very anxious. She saw the accident as unfair, which it was! She was in the right and it shouldn't have happened. However, Paula was able to consider that unfortunately accidents do happen and that some acceptance was needed. Instead, she placed her focus on her recovery.

Tracy was present at an armed robbery. After the robbery she saw the world as very dangerous, didn't think anywhere was safe, and avoided going out. The therapist worked with Tracy to gradually go out to places like a café and the supermarket. Tracy used the coping skills she had learnt to help cope with anxiety in these situations, and was instructed to look out for signs of safety. Tracy learnt that she could focus on the moment and those signs, rather than triggers from the past.

Identify the meaning related to the trauma: The meaning we give to the trauma can keep us stuck.

Eye Movement Desensitization and Reprocessing

This therapy combines exposure with very particular eye movements. It involves being asked to recall aspects of the traumatic event while following particular back-and-forth hand movements by the therapist.

This sounds unusual, but there is good evidence that it helps the brain process the traumatic experiences. A good analogy is that the memories and emotions related to the trauma, which have been constantly active in the mind, are put away in the 'filing cabinet' of memory in our brains.

Trauma-focused Acceptance and Commitment Therapy

As we heard in Chapter 4, this approach focuses on developing our psychological flexibility, and to 'be present, open up, and do what matters'. In trauma it works with our cognitions, including thoughts, images, memories and core beliefs, and with any avoidance or unhelpful patterns of behaviour, such as withdrawing from others or using substances.

Trauma-focused Acceptance and Commitment Therapy uses grounding techniques to help us be present in the moment. It also uses techniques to help us feel comfortable in our bodies, overcome hypervigilance, tolerate distressing feelings and grow self-compassion. It focuses, too, on living a life based on our values, connecting with others, engaging in meaningful activities and setting goals for the future.[24]

More strategies to help with recovery

Hope is a key strategy! Many of these approaches have good evidence for their effectiveness and do help a great deal. Remember, too, that there is a lot to each of us, and we have our personal strengths and resources to draw upon. As hard as trauma is to deal with, we actually learn a great deal about ourselves, and life, through it, and develop more strengths and coping skills.

Hope is key: There are many strategies and approaches that can help.

Remember that relationships can suffer when there has been trauma. Partners or family members may find it helpful to see a doctor or therapist for their own support and assistance, or couples may benefit from relationship counselling (see Chapter 8).

Medication is not often a first-line treatment in trauma. The trauma-focused psychological approaches are tried first. But it may be used if symptoms are severe, or if the person is not benefitting enough from the therapy alone. Medication may also be suggested when psychological treatment is not available, or when the person has a co-existing condition, such as significant depression. Often the selective serotonin reuptake inhibitors (SSRIs) are used (see p. 115). Medication may also be needed to help with nightmares and sleep.

As treatment continues, it is important to see a doctor or therapist to monitor progress. In particular, doctors and therapists will watch out for thoughts of suicide and self-harm.

Narrative Therapy has been used in Australia to assist Aboriginal people, many of whom have experienced significant trauma. This approach, which sees the individual as the expert on themselves and utilizes stories, sits well with Aboriginal people because stories are an integral part of their culture.[25]

Another group who may need specialized assistance is refugees and asylum seekers who have fled their homeland because of war or persecution. They may have experienced significant trauma through separation from family, death of family members, or experiencing abuse or torture. Specialist organizations can assist.

Trauma can involve a great deal of loss and grief, such as loss of loved ones, property or animals. Recovery from loss and grief takes time and a range of emotions can be experienced. Much of what we have talked about will be useful but more information on grief can be found in Chapter 6.

Let's summarize

This chapter has explored the impact of trauma on women. Many of us working in mental health say that if we could change one thing in relation to mental health, it would be preventing various forms of trauma — there would be significantly fewer women experiencing mental health problems.

We looked into the neurobiology of trauma. The nervous system is impacted in different ways by trauma, leading to many of the symptoms we might experience with the acute stress that occurs after a trauma, and the more persistent disorders (post-traumatic stress disorder and complex trauma).

Equally, our neurobiology forms the foundations of treatment, and includes calming activity in certain parts of the brain and activating other parts. An integrated approach, addressing all aspects of ourselves (biological, psychological, social) is a favoured approach. And thanks to neuroplasticity, moving towards healing and flourishing is possible.

Here are the keys from this chapter:

» Bottom-up and top-down approaches involve working with the body to change the brain, and working with the mind, too.

» Working with blame and shame: The perpetrator of abuse and violence is the responsible one. Letting go of self-blame and personal shame is an important part of healing.

» Identify the meaning related to the trauma: The meaning we give to the trauma can keep us stuck.

» Hope is key: There are many strategies and approaches that can help.

11

Managing other issues

"

Not until we are lost do we begin to understand ourselves.

— Henry David Thoreau

The field of mental health is very broad, so it is not possible in this book to cover all the issues that can affect our health. However, in this chapter we will explore a few more, namely:

» addictions, including substance-related issues, gambling and technology

» neurodiversity (autism and attention disorders)

» eating disorders and body image/body dysmorphia

» psychosis

» borderline personality disorder.

These disorders are not necessarily related, and they may appear at different stages in life. Perhaps read the section(s) relevant to you or to loved ones.

Women and addictions

An **addiction** is defined as a strong and compulsive need (i.e. a powerful impulse) to regularly have something (e.g. a drug) or to do something (e.g. to gamble), despite it causing you harm. It results in the inability to stop using the drug or doing the behaviour.

With substances, the word **dependence** is often used rather than addiction, referring to a physical reliance or craving for the substance, resulting in issues such as withdrawal.

The brain responds to a range of experiences (such as eating favourite foods, having sex, getting high on drugs, winning a bet) with pleasure. The brain releases various chemical messengers in the brain, including dopamine, which causes us to feel high. This acts as a reward and we often repeat the behaviour as a result.

Substance-related issues

We have mentioned substance-related issues a few times during the book, in relation to the 'bio-psycho-social' influences on mental health and wellbeing. It is a risk factor for mental health problems, such as depression or non-suicidal self-harm. Substances may be used as a coping strategy for stress, anxiety and depression, grief or loneliness, with unhelpful outcomes such as worsening mood, and it can contribute to anger issues.

A **substance** refers to anything that is used to produce a 'high' or to alter the senses or how alert we are. In our society, we use various drugs for medical reasons and for recreation. Substances used for recreation include alcohol, cannabis, hallucinogens, inhalants, opioids, sedatives and drugs that reduce anxiety, stimulants (such as amphetamine-type substances, cocaine), tobacco and other substances. Many substances create an effect similar to the pleasure response in the brain, releasing chemicals such as dopamine or endorphins (pain-relieving chemicals).

If we become dependent, substance use takes on a life of its own and starts to take over our day-to-day experience. We are at risk of developing mental and behavioural disorders due to substance use and addictive behaviours.

Withdrawal can occur when some drugs are stopped after using them for a long time, causing symptoms such as anxiety, hallucinations or insomnia. Some of these symptoms can be life-threatening.

There are harmful patterns of alcohol use, causing damage to one's physical or mental health, or behaviours leading to the mistreatment of others. And disorders relating to depending on alcohol may include cravings to use alcohol and increasing tolerance to it (needing more of the drug to get the same effect).

Substance-related issues are very common in our communities, and a range of substances are used. Here are a few facts and figures:

» A survey carried out in Australia in 2016 found that about four in ten Australians either smoked daily, drank alcohol in ways that put them at risk of harm, or had used an illicit drug in the previous twelve months.[1]

» Alcohol and tobacco are responsible for 90 per cent of deaths related to substance use.[2]

» Globally, women are reported to consume less alcohol and are two to three times less likely to use an illicit drug than men.

» However, life stage has an impact on use. Women in the middle years are drinking more than 20 years ago, and older women are vulnerable to opioid-based painkillers.[3]

» Women have an 11 per cent lifetime prevalence versus 16 per cent for men in relation to the non-medical use of prescription painkillers.[4]

Substance-related issues and addictions can also be seen as the tip of an iceberg. The substance-related issues sit above the water, and what lies under the water might include factors such as trauma, difficulties coping with feelings, mental health problems, sleep issues, lack of connection with others or struggles with learning or self-worth. The substances may be used to self-medicate and cope.

Many causes or risk factors for the development of substance-related issues have been suggested and include:

» our genetics

» early environmental issues, such as childhood neglect or abuse

» using substances early in life

» social or cultural issues, such as poverty, or having parents or friends who use substances

» having had childhood attention deficit and hyperactivity disorder, or what is called 'conduct disorder' (results in aggression or deceit)

» stresses such as having difficulty expressing feelings or loss and grief

» identifying as gay, transsexual or with another gender or sexual identity

» some physical health problems, such as heart disease, lung disease and chronic pain can trigger substance use

» difficulties coping with various life challenges: for example, not managing at school or at work, or not having activities to do in the community, low self-confidence, lack of supports or lack of coping skills.[5]

Many factors can contribute to substance-related issues, from genetics to various stressors, to lack of support.

Research has shown a number of negative effects of substance use:

» Excessive alcohol increases the risk of injury from accidents and violence.

» Long-term risks from alcohol use include liver and heart disease, cancers and obesity.

» There is a close relationship between substance-related issues and mental illness, and some substances may increase the risk of developing certain mental illnesses.

» Excessive drinking combined with drug use, such as methamphetamines can have very serious legal implications and consequences for our health and safety, or the safety of others.

» E-cigarettes are a relatively new mode of delivering nicotine and their health effects are not yet fully understood.

Unfortunately, we may not recognize that there is a problem, or may not be willing or able to reach out for help. Sometimes we might have to stop and ask ourselves some tough questions, like:

» Am I making excuses for my substance use?

» Am I using substances to forget about my problems?

» Have any financial, legal, medical, family or work problems developed because of using substances?

» Am I in denial about the seriousness of my substance use?

» Am I willing to do almost anything to get hold of the substances?

There are some tools that can help determine whether there is a problem with substance use and whether or not to seek help. The CAGE test and AUDIT questionnaire are examples and are available online.

The aim of treatment is recovery, or the process of improved physical, psychological and social wellbeing and health. And as with other mental health issues and treatments, no 'one size fits all'.

A general approach is harm minimization or reducing the potential harms associated with substance use (e.g. if binge drinking or taking drugs, ensuring a sober friend is around). Here is an example of harm minimization with alcohol:

Verity was experiencing ill-health due to excessive alcohol use. With support, she was able to reduce her alcohol intake from at least one bottle a day to four glasses, then down to two, and finally one glass on most days. Her general health improved as a result.

Recovery from substance-related issues is possible: The aim
of treatment is recovery with improved health and wellbeing.

Motivation is central to getting help and attending treatment.
It is made up of the desire to change, the confidence to do so, and
prioritizing treatment. There is a process in overcoming substance use
that is based on the 'stages of change' model. For example, we may
be at various stages in readiness to quit: we might not be thinking of
quitting at all, or ready to quit and making some plans, or be at the
stage of quitting altogether.

There are approaches that can help. Motivational interviewing, for
example, focuses on identifying any ambivalence about substance use
and harnessing your own resources to change behaviours.

Sometimes it can help to weigh up the pros and cons of using the
substance by making lists. Examples with smoking cigarettes might
be: 'It helps me to relax' (pro) or 'My kids want me to quit' (con). If
relevant, pros or cons could be recorded in your journal.

Here are some strategies to improve motivation:

» Focus on our values and set a goal that fits with these.

» Remember the pros and cons. What will you gain from making
changes?

» Create some new, more helpful habits (see p. 40).

» Acknowledge your success, no matter how small!

» Be aware of unhelpful thoughts or uncomfortable feelings, and
deal with them (see Chapters 4 and 6).

» Get support from others and focus on encouraging thoughts.

» Take action!

Depending on how severe the issues are, a range of treatments may be advised:

» Self-help guides (an example follows).

» Phone-counselling services from local drug and alcohol services.

» Supervised withdrawal programs (at home or in a treatment facility).

» Individual psychological treatment with a therapist, or in a group, exploring the reasons for substance use and how to develop new behaviours and skills.

» Treatment of any related mental health problems.

» Medications to reduce cravings or to replace a dangerous drug with a safer drug, such as opiate substitution programs.

» Lifestyle measures and self-care (see Chapter 2).

» Doing more enjoyable activities that are not related to substance use.

» Maintenance treatment to prevent relapse, such as support groups

» Social supports (such as housing) and growing more social connections.

» Assistance for family or carers.

» Residential rehabilitation.

» Relapse prevention.

Explore the range of treatment options: 'One size does not fit all' and there are a whole range of options, from counselling to residential treatment.

If you are not heavily dependent but want to cut down to safer or less risky levels of drinking, here is an example of a self-help guide for reducing alcohol consumption.

» Monitor — keep a diary of how much and how often you are drinking.

» Change your drinking habits, such as having two drinks instead of four when out, or having non-alcoholic drinks on weekdays.

» Don't drink on an empty stomach.

» Quench thirst with water, rather than alcohol.

» Drink slowly.

» Take a break. Make every second drink a non-alcoholic drink.

» Buy low-alcohol alternatives.

» Avoid salty snacks when drinking (these can make you thirsty and therefore prone to drinking more).

» Do something other than drink.

The above approach may be useful for some women. However, many experiencing substance-related issues grapple with whether they should cease the substance completely or cut down (called 'controlled substance use'). The idea of completely stopping may be too extreme, but they would like to regain control over their substance use.

The more dependent the person is on the substance, the more likely that cutting down or controlled substance use will not be successful. Ceasing completely will then be the best option. It is possible that returning to controlled substance use after a long period of abstinence will be sustainable. However, once a life without substances has been re-established, there is often a reluctance to risk going back to drinking or using, even on rare occasions.

The more dependent on the substance, the more likely that 'controlled substance use' will not be successful. Stopping use completely is likely to be the best option.

There is a range of therapies that can assist. Refer to information on Cognitive Behaviour Therapy in Chapters 4 and 6, and Dialectical Behaviour Therapy in Chapter 7. Behaviours such as staying away from situations associated with substance use are part of therapy. Remember that when the substance is no longer used, cravings or urges will reduce over time. Strategies to cope with cravings can assist:

» Avoid high-risk situations.

» Remove temptations or triggers.

>> The urge to use lasts for short periods of time and will pass. If you have a craving, wait before acting on it. Sit with the urge and use coping skills such as breathing and positive self-talk.

>> Use distraction such as watching a movie or cleaning the house.

>> Remember the 'why', that is, the reason for not using.

>> Call a friend or support agency.

Therapy can also involve noticing our thoughts before using substances (such as 'I can't stand the cravings' or 'A bit won't hurt'). These can then be challenged by asking, 'Is there another way to think about it?' or 'If I am honest with myself, what is the most likely outcome?' Self-critical thoughts, driven by underlying beliefs (such as 'I'm unlovable' or 'I'm a failure') may need to be challenged as well (see p. 61).

Return to the sections about mindfulness and Acceptance and Commitment Therapy in Chapters 4 and 6, to see how they encourage acceptance of thoughts and feelings, no matter how distressing they might be. Substances might seem to help us avoid or numb uncomfortable feelings, but the substances come with negative consequences. The more tools we have to self-soothe, the better (see Chapter 7).

Other addictions

Let's consider two other addictions that may affect mental health and wellbeing, namely gambling and technology use.

Gambling

Only relatively recently has the idea of addiction been applied to problems like gambling, which is common in the western world. The same reward system as in substance use (release of the chemical, dopamine) is switched on in the brain. Gambling and substance use share many features, such as building tolerance, which means increasingly needing to do more of the behaviour to get the same satisfaction. Also, gambling often occurs when there is depression, anxiety or substance-related issues. It can be a way of avoiding uncomfortable feelings and lessening feelings of anxiety or depression.

If gambling is a significant issue, some of the following features will be present:

» Needing to gamble with increasing amounts of money.

» Being restless or irritable when attempting to cut down on gambling.

» Repeatedly failing in efforts to reduce gambling.

» Often being preoccupied with gambling.

» Often gambling when feeling distressed.

» After losing, often returning to chase losses.

» Lying to conceal the extent of gambling.

» Risking or losing significant relationships, jobs or educational opportunities.

» Relying on other people to provide money because of financial problems.[6]

Gambling can have a major effect on relationships, families, work and finances, as well as on our sense of self-worth and mental health. It is important to recognize that there is a problem and to ask for help.

There are organizations in the community and professionals with expertise that can assist. There can be a lot of shame and stigma to overcome in reaching out, and it is vital to treat any related trauma, depression or anxiety.

Gambling can have major effects on all aspects of life. It is vital to recognize that there is a problem and ask for help.

There are self-help resources available, and it can be useful to join a support group. Increasing social connections and supports is recommended, along with doing more activities that relieve stress. Getting rid of credit cards and seeking financial counselling may assist.

Depending on the individual, the focus may be on behaviours related to seeking pleasure, on beliefs around being able to control random events, or exposing particular cues related to gambling (such as the sounds or visual cues of slot machines) to lessen the urge to gamble. The strategies to manage urges covered in the last section on substance use may assist. Postponing gambling, distraction and using relaxation techniques are recommended. Part of recovery is learning to manage uncomfortable emotions (see p. 36).

Technology

Technology is fabulous, but it is a problem when there is compulsive use. Research suggests that many people spend more than 46 hours per week looking at screens and, on average, check their smartphones about 85 times a day.[7] The fact that tablets or smartphones can be taken anywhere means that compulsions can readily be acted on. Again, the release of dopamine in the brain is related to technology use, and tolerance can be developed so that increasing amounts of time on the device are needed to give the same pleasure response.

The name for smartphone addiction is nomophobia, the fear of being without a mobile device or smartphone.

Technology addiction may be related to:

» virtual relationships via social media, dating apps, texting or messaging, rather than having relationships with real people

» compulsive web searching, watching videos or checking sites, causing us to neglect other aspects of our life

» cybersex addiction with hours spent on sexting or adult-messaging, impacting negatively on life

» online compulsions such as gaming or shopping, which can cause many financial or social issues.[8]

It can result in:

» worsening stress, anxiety, loneliness and depression

» reduced attention and concentration due to the constant stream of stimulation overwhelming the brain

» reduced ability to think deeply or creatively, to remember and learn

» sleep disturbances

» being more self-absorbed.

Signs of being addicted to technology include sneaking off to use a device, lying about how much time is being spent using it, getting irritable when interrupted, or feeling panicky the smartphone or device has been left somewhere and we are without it. Another sign is 'fear of missing out' (FOMO) on something that's going on online, which has become pervasive in society.

So, what are the options for managing a technology addiction?

» Get support from family, friends or a therapist.

» Recognize the triggers such as boredom, stress or feeling low.

» Get treatment for any underlying issues, such as depression or trauma.

» Set a goal to cut back using the device and use your journal to keep a record of use.

» Regularly turn off the device and adopt device-free places in the home and car.

» Work on your coping skills (e.g. managing stress, sitting with uncomfortable emotions (see Chapters 4 and 7)).

» Replace device use with other activities, such as reading or exercise.

» Accept that you can't keep up with everything that's going on online.

» Remove some social media apps.

> » Find people to interact with face to face.
>
> » And don't forget that children imitate us, so be a role model to them!
>
> » If you need assistance, consider seeing a therapist or seek out a support group.

Deal with technology addiction: By recognizing that there is a problem and getting some support. Focus on other activities and interacting with people face to face.

Borderline personality disorder

Borderline personality disorder is a long-term mental disorder that affects interpersonal relationships, mood and behaviour. There may be traits of the disorder, or symptoms that don't cause major issues, or a disorder, which is more severe.

When the disorder is present, there is often struggle with self-identity or having a sense of who you are, difficulty in regulating emotions (with outbursts of crying or anger) and impulsive and self-sabotaging behaviours. Self-harming behaviours can occur. It is characterized by fear of abandonment and having unstable relationships.

There may be a genetic tendency to the condition, and there might be a history of abuse or trauma related to attachment to caregivers (see

p. 241). The latter has occurred in approximately 40 to 70 per cent of those with this disorder.[9] There are often co-existing issues such as depression, bipolar disorder, anxiety, addictions, eating disorders or psychosis.

There can be stigma about the disorder, making it harder to access support or treatment. However, treatment can assist greatly, and the focus is on creating a more stable, internalized sense of self, and learning emotion regulation, cognitive and interpersonal skills (such as through Dialectical Behaviour Therapy). Various medications may be needed, especially when other conditions are present.

It can be very hard to differentiate borderline personality disorder from complex post-traumatic stress disorder, which we looked at in Chapter 10. There is overlap but the main differences relate to the fear of abandonment and more frequent self-harming behaviours in borderline personality disorder.[10]

In borderline personality disorder there is a fear of abandonment and self-harming behaviours, along with difficulties managing emotions and relationships.

Neurodiversity

Autism and attention disorders are part of what is called 'neurodiversity'. This means there are variations between people in the development of their nervous system, including the brain. In fact, we all have diverse brains, and with autism there can be a very wide range of variations (from mild symptoms to those which are very severe and disabling). We are going to look at autism and attention disorders, and these may occur together.

Autism

Autism often becomes evident in the early years of life, and it persists into adulthood. However, many women are not diagnosed in childhood, and may seek help in adulthood. Diagnosis can explain symptoms and challenges that may have been experienced earlier in life, and this on its own can be helpful.

Autism is characterized by difficulties in communication (language, and also social and non-verbal cues), and repetitive patterns of behaviour or interests, which possibly occur to distract the person from distressing symptoms, such as anxiety. Sensory issues can also occur, creating intolerance of various sensations such as certain clothing touching the skin or eating certain foods. Behaviours such as rocking may occur to block out other sensory input being experienced as disturbing.

There are various theories about why it occurs, including our genetics, parents being older in age, and environmental factors triggering a tendency to autism.[11] A thorough assessment is needed to identify autism, including related issues, as mental health issues such as anxiety, mood, attention and psychotic disorders are more frequent. Autistic people more commonly identify as part of the LGBTIQA+ community.[12]

A range of treatment and support options are available for autistic adults, including education about autism, behavioural therapy, social skills training, life skills coaching, communication skills training and psychological or medical therapies for anxiety and depression. Family or carers may need support.

Attention disorders

Women of all age groups can be affected by attention disorders, in which there can be difficulties with getting started on tasks, keeping attention on the task at hand and avoiding distraction, remembering to do things or losing things, being impulsive (acting without thinking things through), planning and organizing, being on time and managing emotions, such as frustration and boredom.

These difficulties are thought to be related to lowered levels of the chemical messenger dopamine in particular parts of the brain. Dopamine helps us give attention to tasks. By adulthood, some of these behaviours might be less of a problem, might occur in different ways, or other difficulties might become more apparent. For example, there may still be struggle with maintaining attention, remembering instructions, managing time and finishing tasks.

Difficulties regulating emotions may also occur, resulting in feeling overwhelmed, having angry outbursts, feeling socially anxious or developing low self-worth. All these difficulties can result in challenges with education, achieving life goals or having performance issues at work. There may also be difficulties maintaining relationships or financial difficulties due to impulsive spending. There can be legal consequences secondary to impulsive behaviours, and this is more likely if there are associated substance use issues.

Assessment of attention disorders is important: Even though there is a lot of information online about attention disorders, it is vital to have a thorough assessment by experienced professionals.

There are many treatment options available, including education about attention issues, addressing lifestyle (such as regular sleep, exercise and healthy foods), assistance with aspects such as sleep problems and various approaches, such as regulating attention, communication skills, time management and emotional regulation to manage frustration.

It is also important to work on self-belief and self-confidence as these have often been eroded through life experiences, and to deal with any risk-taking behaviours or addictions. Online forums or support groups may help. And medication may be suggested. This includes stimulant drugs to increase dopamine levels.

Authors Greg Crosby and Tonya Lippert say that the problem with attention disorders is regulating attention, rather than a lack of attention. This means there is a struggle to focus on more mundane activities and a bias towards very stimulating activities (which trigger more dopamine release. The authors suggest learning skills to regulate action and attention, such as minimizing distractions and using reminders for activities (lists, planners or alarms), breaking tasks down into chunks and using a reward when activities are completed. Mindfulness can also help.[13]

Eating disorders

Eating disorders are psychological and medical disorders that involve over-evaluation of body shape and weight and over-investment in controlling shape and weight. There are serious abnormalities in eating and weight control behaviours. Women of all ages can be impacted by eating disorders. Unfortunately, they can become chronic and some people will die due to the eating disorder.

Eating disorders have become a major health problem across the world, predominantly affecting women. The prevalence in Australia is about 9 per cent of the adult population, and this figure continues to increase. Some studies report a prevalence as high as 16.3 per cent in older adolescents and adults. More people die from anorexia than all other psychiatric disorders (20 per cent).[14]

The most common eating disorders are **anorexia nervosa**, which is a refusal to maintain a minimally normal body weight, and **bulimia nervosa**, which refers to repeated episodes of binge eating followed by inappropriate compensatory behaviours such as vomiting, misuse of laxatives, diuretics or other medications, fasting or excessive exercise. There are a number of other eating disorders such as night eating syndrome.[15]

A disturbance in the perception of body shape and weight is an essential feature of both anorexia and bulimia, and remember that weight can still be normal with an eating disorder. Also, we might begin with one eating disorder and move over time to another, such as being impacted by anorexia and later bulimia.

Eating disorders involve over-evaluation and control of body shape and weight. There is a disturbance in perception of body shape and weight.

Eating disorders are thought to result from a whole range of factors, including genetic vulnerability, stage of development (more at risk in adolescence), personality style (being a perfectionist or having obsessional tendencies), relationship and family problems, and the influences of society and culture. We receive messages about our bodies throughout our lives, from others and via media. Related to this, there may be significant body image issues (see next section).

Despite the seriousness of many of the symptoms of eating disorders, there may be denial that there is a problem. However, early identification is important. Other mental health problems may be present, such as anxiety and depression, post-traumatic stress disorder, borderline personality disorder or autism.

Different signs and symptoms may be noticed, such as:

» using food as way to control or express emotions

» obsessional eating behaviours or increased exercise

» thinking about food, weight and body appearance a lot

» feeling scared about gaining weight

» withdrawing from family and friends

» difficulties sleeping or concentrating on studies or at work

» irritability

» reduced energy

» lowered self-confidence

» low mood or anxiety symptoms

» possibly self-harm and suicidal thinking.

The SCOFF questionnaire is a basic screening tool for eating disorders. It can be used when there is concern that an eating disorder might exist rather than to make a diagnosis. It asks a series of questions, and a score of 2 or more 'yes' responses raises suspicion of an eating disorder:

» **S:** Do you make yourself sick because you feel uncomfortably full?

» **C:** Do you worry you have lost control over how much you eat?

» **O:** Have you recently lost more than one stone (6.35 kg) in a three-month period?

» **F:** Do you believe yourself to be fat when others say you are too thin?

» **F:** Would you say food dominates your life?

An answer of 'yes' to two or more questions warrants further questioning and more comprehensive assessment. A further two questions have been shown to indicate a high likelihood of bulimia nervosa, namely: 'Are you satisfied with your eating patterns? Do you ever eat in secret?'[16]

A thorough medical assessment (including blood tests) is needed to assess nutritional status and vital signs such as blood pressure. When there are concerns about physical safety, a hospital admission may be required to medically stabilize the person and reverse the effects of starvation.

A non-blaming approach is essential, and a psychological and possibly psychiatric assessment may also be needed. Talking therapies may include Cognitive Behaviour Therapy (adapted for eating disorders), Acceptance and Commitment Therapy, Dialectical Behaviour Therapy, Interpersonal Therapy and Narrative Therapy. There is also the 'Maudsley model of therapy for adults with anorexia nervosa'.

Holistic treatment is vital: Non-blaming, holistic and team-based care is needed to address the biological, psychological and social aspects of eating disorders. Self-compassion is vital.

Treatment generally involves:

» a team approach, with a nutritionist, therapist, and doctor(s)

» education about eating disorders

» self-help programs if the issues are mild

» ongoing medical checks

» regular talking therapy

» working on self-confidence and social skills, such as assertiveness

» practising more self-compassion (see p. 49)

» teaching coping skills and emotion regulation (see Chapter 7)

» addressing body image issues and dissatisfaction

» addressing perfectionism

» treatment of related mental health problems

» possibly medication

» hospital programs if the issues are more severe

» outpatient treatment programs at specialized centres

» support for family and carers

» fostering hope.

For family member, friends or carers who are worried about a woman who may have an eating disorder, aim to help her feel safe in talking about the issues. Be supportive and if they don't wish to talk with you, help them to find someone they can talk to. Learn about eating disorders beforehand and choose a private place to chat. Be kind and empathetic and discuss your concerns.

Here are some tips from Mental Health First Aid Australia about when to seek urgent assistance:

» if non-suicidal self-harming behaviours or suicidal thoughts are present

» if weight is low or has dropped suddenly, or eating patterns have changed suddenly

» if the woman is confused or disoriented

» if there are fainting spells, or they are feeling very cold or weak

» if there are painful muscle spasms or an irregular heartbeat

» if they are having chest pain or trouble breathing.[17]

Body image issues and body dysmorphia

Body image refers to how we think, feel and behave in relation to physical appearance.[18] It's normal to have moments where we may feel dissatisfied, unhappy or uncomfortable in our own body. But if these feelings intensify, a more serious issue may be developing, and we may become more at risk of engaging in unhealthy and unhelpful behaviours around food, exercise and supplements — all of which can impact on our mental and physical health.

Poor body image can lead to:

» low self-belief

» obsessively thinking about the body and appearance

» putting too much emphasis on weight, shape or size

» frequently comparing our body and appearance with other people

» changes to eating and exercise behaviours in an attempt to change our weight or muscularity

» withdrawing from things usually enjoyed, like sports and social activities

» relationship changes with friends, family members and partners

» other mental health concerns such as depression or anxiety

» engaging in risky behaviours, such as smoking, abusing substances or increased sexual activity.[19]

Body dysmorphia is a separate disorder that involves preoccupation with one or more features of the body that are either not present or only slightly present.[20] This leads to a great deal of anxiety, frequent checking of appearance and seeking reassurance, and possibly skin picking. It can be associated with having cosmetic procedures that are not needed, excess exercise and possibly eating disorders.

There can be significant issues with self-worth, body image and shame with this disorder. Thinking and behaviours are often obsessional, and anxiety and depression, or suicidal thinking can result.

Body image refers to how we feel about our appearance. Body dysmorphia involves preoccupation with feature(s) of the body that are not, or only slightly, present.

A range of treatments are available, including education and support, improving self-belief (see Chapter 3), talking therapies such as Cognitive Behaviour Therapy, managing the anxiety and depression (see Chapters 4 and 6), learning more coping and emotion regulation skills (see Chapter 7), and medication if needed. It is important for family and doctors to be understanding and supportive, but not support the false belief about the body.

In relation to body image issues and body dysmorphia, it can help to:

» understand society's influence and unrealistic ideals that are promoted (mostly to sell something)

» reduce exposure to images for flawless beauty, fitness or appearance; remember photos on social media or in magazines are manipulated and photoshopped

» drop comparisons with other people

» recognize that we are amazing, including our bodies, and that we are a whole person with many different aspects to ourselves

>> look after our bodies and focus on eating and exercise for health and wellbeing

>> be grateful for our bodies

>> not participate in buying diet products

>> focus on the parts of ourselves that we do like

>> avoid trying to look like someone else

>> remember our strengths and resources

>> challenge or let go of unhelpful and self-critical thoughts

>> practise self-care and self-compassion.[21]

To improve body image: Drop comparisons and self-criticism, reduce time on social media, and know that we are more than our bodies and have many strengths.

Psychosis

The term **psychosis** refers to losing contact with reality. There are many causes of psychosis, but the main ones are schizophrenia and drug-induced psychosis. Schizophrenia has a usual onset in the early 20s and is mostly a long-term issue.

There can be high levels of depression and loss of social functioning with schizophrenia; however, it is treatable and many people lead fulfilling lives. Drug-induced psychosis is due to recreational drugs (hallucinogens, amphetamines, stimulants) and mostly stops when the drugs are gone.

The main symptoms of psychosis are:

» changes in emotion and motivation (depression, anxiety, irritability, suspiciousness, blunted emotion, reduced motivation)

» changes in thinking and perception, including reduced concentration, interrupted trains of thought, a sense of alteration of self or others, fixed ideas that are unusual (e.g. people conspiring against us), or hallucinations (often auditory, i.e. hearing things that are not real, or visual, i.e. seeing things that are not present)

» changes to behaviour, such as sleep disturbances, social isolation or agitation.

The treatment of psychosis involves:

» early intervention and taking a holistic approach

» having a comprehensive treatment plan

» education about the condition and treatments

» support

» improving lifestyle, including diet, exercise, sleep and activity levels

» managing stress

» talking therapies

» working with loss and grief, and sense of self-worth and identity

» working closely with families

» group programs for education, support and skills training

» fostering involvement in the community

» assistance with housing, finances

» treatment of associated issues, such as depression or substance use

» monitoring physical health and wellbeing

» maintaining hope and focusing on recovery

» having a relapse prevention plan (see p. 159)

» suicide prevention strategies

» medication (antipsychotics, mood stabilizers)

» support for families or carers.

Early treatment in psychosis is vital and improves outcomes. Seek help early.

If concerned about a loved one with psychosis, the mental health first aid involves being empathetic and speaking to them privately about their experiences. It is important not to be confrontational and to communicate in a clear way. Focus on listening and on letting them know that there is professional help available.[22] There is greater risk of self-harm and suicide when psychosis is present, so refer to Chapter 7 about how to respond.

At times the person with psychosis will be compulsorily detained (or sectioned) at a hospital for assessment and treatment. This occurs when the person is a risk to themselves or another person and needs immediate treatment. Detention occurs when the person does not agree to be voluntarily admitted. The aim is to ensure the person is safe and receives the treatment they need.

 ## Let's summarize

Some of the issues raised in this chapter need a thorough and early assessment when there are concerns. It is important to ensure the issue is identified and appropriate treatment can be considered. Understanding the disorder(s) and having a thorough treatment plan are vital.

Exploring underlying reasons for mental health issues and addressing these, plus having a range of coping strategies is vital. There are specific therapies that have been developed for particular disorders, and finding therapists skilled with these is important. Maintaining hope and focusing on recovery are central. A summary of the keys is provided:

» Recovery from substance-related issues is possible.

» Explore the range of treatment options, as 'one size does not fit all'.

» Deal with technology addiction by recognizing there is a problem and getting some support.

» Assessment of attention disorders is important.

» Holistic treatment is vital for eating disorders.

» To improve body image, drop comparisons and self-criticism, reduce time on social media, and know that we are more than our bodies and have many strengths.

12

Navigating later life

This chapter explores our mental health and wellbeing in later life. We talk about the late phase of life being from 60 years of age on. We will look at ageing, with a focus on 'positive ageing', and consider some mental health issues that might occur during this phase of life.

We will also consider the impact of chronic illness, cancer and pain on mental health and wellbeing, and approaches that may assist. Dementia will be covered, too.

Ageing

It is worth mentioning a couple of figures at the outset. Life expectancy (or how long a person is expected to live on average) for women has steadily increased over the years. Current expectancies in the western world for women sit around 85 years of age. And the population is ageing rapidly. Between 2015 and 2050 the proportion of the world's population over 60 will go from 12 per cent to 22 per cent.[1]

From 60 years of age there is much change in our lives, often rewarding and sometimes challenging. There is the possiblity of retirement, enjoying activities such as travel and connections with grandchildren, and moving to a smaller house and more. There are physical changes, and as time goes on possibly health issues, or loss of loved ones.

There are also age-related changes to our cognitive abilities too, with changes to reaction times, difficulties learning new material or with our recall or day-to-day memory. However, we do bring in our knowledge from experience to assist.

Common challenges during this life stage include:

» maintaining health and fitness

» maintaining social networks and activities

» feelings of sadness and loss

» ensuring financial security

» decreases in mobility

» frailty and an increased reliance on others.[2]

The term 'positive ageing' is helpful. It refers to the process of maintaining a positive attitude, keeping fit and healthy, and engaging fully in life as we grow older.[3] We know about some of the factors that contribute to positive ageing. For example, exercise contributes to physical and mental health. And research has shown that having a sense of life satisfaction is associated with health benefits and living longer.[4] Spirituality and religiosity also contribute positively to ageing and wellbeing, through connection and involvement with others and meaningful activities, and personal growth.[5]

Positive ageing is about maintaining a positive attitude and engaging fully in life. It includes our mental health and wellbeing and sounds very much like flourishing!

Health and wellbeing in older adults is influenced by an interaction of environmental, psychological, spiritual and genetic factors. It makes sense, then, that to foster positive ageing we can adopt a range of strategies:

» Eating a healthy diet.

» Keeping moving (gardening, exercise).

» Avoiding alcohol and smoking.

» Staying hydrated.

» Having more positive ideas and beliefs about ageing.

» Maintaining a positive attitude to ourselves and life.

» Reframing negative thinking (see p. 102).

» Adapting to change (see Chapter 5).

» Staying connected — *quality* relationships are key (see p. 186).

» Having a routine.

» Having a sense of purpose and meaning (see p. 51).

» Keeping your brain active (e.g. part-time employment or courses).

» Managing stress (see Chapter 4).

» Getting good sleep.

» Practising gratitude.

» Helping others.

» Having regular medical check-ups.

» Having a regular laugh.

Note that a number of these can help with adapting to retirement as well, especially staying connected, having a routine and finding a sense of purpose.

Foster positive ageing: Through a healthy lifestyle, positive attitudes, purpose, staying connected and laughter!

Depression

Around 15 per cent of adults over 60 suffer from a mental disorder, and about 20 per cent of older people have mild but significant depressive symptoms (1.23 per cent fulfil the criteria of depression).[6]

We tend to do a **life review** as we get older. This can lead to being satisfied with what we have achieved and concluding that we have had a good life, or alternatively thinking that we haven't achieved what we wanted. The former can lead to acceptance and contentment (Kahlil Gibran summed this up: 'To be able to look back upon one's life in satisfaction, is to live twice'), whereas the latter can lead to feeling depressed.

Depression may also be related to the challenges mentioned earlier and the associated loss and grief. The symptoms may not be as obvious as in younger people, and there may be a focus on physical symptoms such as tiredness or lack of energy. It is important to see a doctor to exclude any physical causes, and to assess for dementia as the symptoms overlap.

Let's hear about Sylvia, 75 years of age and feeling low in mood:

Sylvia lives with her husband John, who has dementia. She finished work when she was 68 and they travelled for a few years before John was diagnosed. They don't travel any more due to the dementia.

Sylvia finds herself feeling tired and low in mood. She feels guilty when she is irritable with John, but she doesn't quite know what to do about this. On top of this her arthritis has got worse, and her daughter isn't visiting very often any more.

Sylvia's mood was depressed, but there wasn't a diagnosis of depression at this stage. We will hear more about her later in the chapter. With depression, many of the strategies outlined in Chapter 4, including talking therapies, will assist.

Elder abuse

It is important to be aware of the possibility of elder abuse, which is thought to affect up to 5 per cent of older people and may contribute to anxiety or depression.[7] This includes 'any deliberate or unintentional action, or lack of action, carried out by a person in a trusted relationship, which causes distress, harm, or serious risk of harm to an older person, or loss or damage to property or assets'.[8]

Elder abuse may involve physical, psychological, social, sexual or financial abuse, or involve neglect or misuse of medicines (withholding or overuse). It is more likely to be carried out by a relative such as a son or daughter, spouse or domestic partner, grandchild, friend or neighbour, or paid or unpaid carer. However, we all have rights, including safety, and support can be gained from a doctor and abuse reported to police.

Chronic illness, cancer and pain

It is important to remember that growing older does not have to mean growing sicker. It is reported that 80 per cent of the chronic diseases of ageing, and the biggest cause of poor health in older women, are preventable, and that looking after our physical and mental health and wellbeing needs to be a focus from midlife as a way of preventing chronic illnesses.[9]

Chronic disease

Chronic diseases are prolonged physical or mental illnesses that are often not cured completely.[10] Women may be impacted by heart or lung disease, osteoporosis or diabetes, or myalgic encephalomyelitis–chronic fatigue (ME/CFS). Depression and arthritis affect more older women than men, and can significantly impact quality of life. Dementia is considered a chronic disease, too, and we will consider it in a moment.

These diseases may be influenced by genetics and lifestyle, including what we eat and drink, and exercise. We need a healthy body to have a healthy brain, and recent evidence suggests that inflammation (the body's reaction to infection or injury) may lead to organ damage. With chronic illness we may have a low-grade inflammation over many years, and it is also thought that inflammation may be linked with dementia or depression.[11]

Mental and physical health are inter-related, and mental illness can impact physical health and wellbeing. For example, depression is associated with physical inactivity, weight gain, diabetes and heart disease. Schizophrenia is associated with increased smoking, weight gain and chronic illness, such as diabetes and lung disease. In relation to this, we need to reduce risk factors such as smoking and poverty, and grow the protective factors such as healthy lifestyle and regular health checks. Good psychosocial support is vital, too, as are effective treatment of mental health disorders and encouragement of self-management.

When we develop a chronic illness we need to adapt and use our coping skills. Sometimes we might deny there is an issue or divert our feelings into harmful activities.

Having information and support can assist with adapting, and there may be a need for practical assistance in terms of financial issues or day-to-day functioning. Our self-worth or sense of identity may be challenged, and support in dealing with this, along with any impacts on relationships or sexuality, is vital. Goals may need to be adjusted, and maintaining connection and meaningful activity are important.

Talking therapies may be of assistance, as there may be a sense of loss and grief (see Chapter 7). Anxiety or depression may also be present, so working on helpful thoughts and behaviours can assist. Having routine and positive habits (such as exercise or meditation) and developing more optimistic thinking can aid adapting and wellbeing. Coming to an acceptance of the illness is part of adaptation.[12]

Foster wellbeing in chronic disease: Many approaches can help, such as having routine and working on a healthy lifestyle and helpful thinking.

Cancer

Cancer can have a profound impact on our mental health and wellbeing. The diagnosis can cause significant emotional distress and potentially trauma. There may be shock, denial, anger or sadness. Symptoms of anxiety, depression (reported in 30 to 40 per cent) or post-traumatic stress disorder may arise.[13] The medical treatment may be traumatic, and chemotherapy or hormonal therapy may impact mood, sleep and memory.

With improved treatments in recent years for many cancers, many women are surviving cancer. This is wonderful, but we need to remember that there can be many issues to cope with, such as the impact of ongoing treatments, impact on relationships, dealing with survivor guilt or fear of recurrence. Much of the discussion about adaptation in relation to chronic illness applies, and it is vital that appropriate support is sought and provided.

Pain

Pain is defined as 'an unpleasant sensory and emotional experience associated with actual or potential tissue damage'.[14] Pain is complex, and it is experienced both physically and emotionally. About 20 per cent of us will experience **chronic pain**, or pain lasting more than a few months.[15]

Strategies to assist with chronic pain include:

 » education

 » a holistic approach

» having a support team (family and friends, carers, health professionals such as doctor, physiotherapist, psychologist, pain specialist)

» getting good quality sleep

» having as healthy a lifestyle as possible, including exercise

» setting small goals

» living a life consistent with our values

» managing stress

» breathing and relaxation techniques, meditation

» staying away from substance use

» planning days and pacing activity (avoiding overdoing things and then 'crashing')

» having things to look forward and scheduling some pleasurable activities

» staying connected with people

» therapies such as Cognitive Behavioural Therapy, biofeedback and mindfulness-based treatment

» practical help with the household chores and shopping

» appropriate medication

» pain clinics (nerve blocks or devices)

» practising self-compassion.

Many strategies can help with chronic pain: A holistic approach can help, along with practical support and various therapies.

Dementia is a term for a group of disorders affecting the brain. It describes a collection of symptoms for which the cause can vary greatly. Dementia mostly affects older women, but it can occur earlier. It is a common cause of hospital admissions and death in older people throughout the world. About 60 million people worldwide have dementia, but these numbers are rising.[16]

Dementia mainly affects older people, but it is not a normal part of ageing.

The most common types of dementia are Alzheimer's disease, vascular dementia (due to problems with blood flow in the brain), Lewy body disease (loss of nerve cells in the brain due to abnormal protein deposits called 'Lewy bodies'), frontotemporal dementia (referring to particular parts of the brain that deteriorate), and alcohol-related dementia.

The early signs of dementia include memory loss (progressive or frequent), confusion, personality change, apathy and withdrawing socially, and loss of ability to perform everyday tasks.

It is important to have a careful assessment by your doctor or a geriatrician, as some medical conditions can mimic dementia (e.g. depression, low thyroid, some vitamin deficiencies, over-medication, brain tumours).

The treatment of dementia includes:

» education about dementia and its management

» support groups

» counselling, including for the family

» working through loss and grief

» stimulating cognition (memory, attention) and activity

» practical guidance about planning ahead about money and advanced care directives

» strategies for reducing stress and anxiety

» improving lifestyle

» regular health checks

» drug treatments to slow the progression of the dementia

» treating related symptoms (such as depression or hearing loss)

» support for family or carers, including online forums, seeing a therapist or respite.

Remember Sylvia from earlier in the chapter?

Sylvia was contending with changes in later life, being a carer and feeling more isolated. John had issues related to the dementia. Caring for both John and his carer is vital. Seeing a doctor and a therapist helped Sylvia work through the issues and her feelings, including speaking with her daughter, and organizing more practical support.

Refer, too, to the section on burnout, which can apply to carers, on p. 126.

> **The treatment of dementia:** Includes education and support, for the person and their carers. Healthy lifestyle and medication may assist.

Let's summarize

Biological ageing is inevitable, but we can make choices across our lifespan to prevent illness and promote 'positive ageing'. Taking a bio-psycho-social approach to maintaining our mental health and wellbeing is important, as are our attitude and having a healthy lifestyle.

When there is chronic disease, cancer or pain impacting us, having support and talking through issues can help. Adaptation is needed, and various coping skills can help. Sometimes acceptance needs to be fostered. A holistic approach is always best.

The keys from the chapter are summarized here:

» Foster positive ageing through a healthy lifestyle, positive attitudes, purpose, staying connected and laughter!

» Foster wellbeing in chronic disease by having routine and working on a healthy lifestyle and helpful thinking.

» Many strategies can help with chronic pain, and a holistic approach can help.

» The treatment of dementia includes education and support, for the person and their carers.

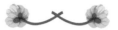

Final words on flourishing

> **"**
>
> Follow your bliss and the universe will open doors
> where there were only walls.
>
> — Joseph Campbell

Let's go back to the start of the book and reflect for a few moments. The first paragraph says that flourishing is all about thriving in life and is strongly influenced by our mental health and wellbeing. It also says that, at times, it is very hard to have a sense of flourishing, especially when life throws challenges in our path.

This set the scene for the book, as we have times of great joy and times with great challenges in life, such as the pandemic or dealing with a mental health issue. Supported by evidence of the importance of addressing mental wellbeing alongside any mental health issues, we have taken an 'and-both' approach and explored ways to work with both. At the core of the book has been the aim of flourishing.

Often, challenges are due to change, and we are constantly adapting as we travel through life. We need strategies to be able to adapt, and so in the book we have highlighted many doors and keys. The doors have represented important information to be aware of, and the keys have involved practical strategies to help us move towards wellbeing and flourishing.

In the first chapter, we looked at information about women and mental health, and why we tend to put ourselves last. Several important points became evident. As a society we need to address issues such as poverty, homelessness and trauma. And as individuals we need to prioritize ourselves and our mental health and wellbeing, including self-care.

In Chapter 2 we identified ten foundational steps to help us improve our mental health and wellbeing. These steps can be helpful whether or not there are mental health issues, and can be individualized to meet our own needs. In a way, they operate as a mental health check too, as they remind us to reflect on where we might be up to with the various steps.

The steps are:

1. Raise self-awareness and identify what to focus on.

2. Be mindful of your emotions.

3. Choose some intentions or goals.

4. Attend to physical health, lifestyle and self-care.

5. Connect with others.

6. Tap into talking therapies (to manage thoughts, feelings and behaviours).

7. Know and use your strengths.

8. Explore self-compassion, meaning and purpose.

9. Enjoy meaningful activities and practise gratitude.

10. Consider complementary therapies or medication if needed (for mental health issues).

There was a prevention focus, too, including fostering mindfulness and a growth mindset. Our brains are truly amazing and due to neuroplasticity they can change, hence all of the information and practical strategies to foster new connections within the brain.

We went on to tackle self-belief, managing stress and anxiety, adapting to change and challenges (including burnout), depression and loss and grief. Many helpful approaches and strategies were shared, such as reframing or defusing thoughts, relaxation and mindfulness techniques, and changing our story.

We have a whole range of emotions, some of which feel fabulous, and some which are distressing. In Chapter 7 we focused on ways to sit with uncomfortable feelings, tolerate distress and soothe ourselves. And Chapters 8 and 9 delved into particular topics that can be of concern to women, namely hormonal and reproductive issues and relationships.

Chapter 10 was particularly important as it explores trauma and its impacts. The statistics about women and trauma are awful, and talking more about this may contribute to making a difference in society and for individual women. In Chapters 11 and 12 we explored other mental health issues affecting women, and the later stage of life and 'positive ageing'.

As we have worked through the chapters, we have naturally

considered how we are tracking in different areas of our lives, and perhaps on our sense of life satisfaction. COVID-19 has definitely impacted us. Levels of stress and various mental health problems have increased. Despite this, it has been an opportunity to evaluate our lives, and what is important to us, and perhaps make some important changes.

There has been a great deal of learning during *The Flourishing Woman*. One strategy has been kept until now. We are almost 'home' in terms of the book, and when we are feeling stressed, we can also think of HOME:

» **H**ope: learn from what is happening.

» **O**pportunity: grow from what we are learning.

» **M**ake change: either the situation or our response to it.

» **E**ngage help: connect with others and ask for support.[1]

It has been a joy travelling with you through *The Flourishing Woman*. A final question comes to mind: 'What are the final words that stand out from nearly 350 pages?' We will all have different ideas, but maybe:

» Enough.

» Strengths and values.

» Positive emotions like gratitude.

» Meaningful activities and purpose.

» Connection and belonging.

» Mindfulness and self-compassion.

» Courage.

» Learning and practice (and more practice).

» Always hope, love and laughter!

To finish, Marianne Williamson wrote: 'Our deepest fear is not that we are inadequate. Our deepest fear is that we are powerful beyond measure. It is our light, not our darkness, that most frightens us.' She went on to write: 'As we let our own light shine, we unconsciously give other people the permission to do the same'.[2]

My hope is that this book has provided numerous keys and opened many doors related to growth, change, opportunity, healing, self-compassion and potential. Maybe it has opened a particular door, one that gives us permission for our light to shine ... as we become, or continue to be, flourishing women.

Resources

Acceptance and Commitment Therapy: www.actmindfully.com.au

Anxiety Australia: https://thiswayup.org.au/

Anxiety UK: www.anxietyuk.org.uk

Anxiety USA: www.anxiety.org

Australasian Menopause Society: www.menopause.org.au/

Black Dog Institute: www.blackdoginstitute.org.au

Blue Pages (depression): www.bluepages.anu.edu.au

Butterfly Foundation (eating disorders): https://butterfly.org.au/

Centre for Clinical Interventions: www.cci.health.wa.gov.au

Dementia: www.dementia.org

GriefLink (grief and suicide information):
    https://grieflink.org.au/factsheets/grief-and-suicide/

Kesler-10 Scale: www.blackdoginstitute.org.au/wp-content/
    uploads/2020/04/k10.pdf

Mental Health Foundation UK: www.mentalhealth.org.uk

Mental Health Foundation of New Zealand: www.mentalhealth.org.nz

Mental health and wellbeing resources: www.drcatehowell.com.au

Mental Health First Aid Australia: www.mhfa.com.au

Moodgym (online treatment program for depression): https://moodgym.anu.edu.au

National Council on Problem Gambling: www.ncpgambling.org/programs-resources/

NZ Drug Foundation: www.drugfoundation.org.nz

Perimenopause depression assessment tool: www.menopausecbtclinic. co.uk/wp-content/uploads/2020/11/MENO-D.pdf

Australian Psychological Society: www.psychology.org.au

American Psychological Association: www.apa.org

Psychology Today: www.psychologytoday.com

Smiling Mind (mindfulness app): www.smilingmind.com.au

Strengths questionnaire: www.viacharacter.org/character-strengths-via

Phoenix Australia, trauma information: www.phoenixaustralia.org/about/

Endnotes

Introduction

1. Iasiello, M., Van Agteren, J. and Cochrane, E.M. 2020, 'Mental health and/or mental illness: A scoping review of the evidence and implications of the dual-continua model of mental health', *Evidence Base*, (1), pp. 1–45.

2. McKay, S. 2018, *The Women's Brain Book: The neuroscience of health, hormones and happiness*, Hachette Australia, Sydney, p. 31.

3. Burrowed, K. 2021, 'Gender bias is still putting women's health at risk', retrieved from www1.racgp.org.au/newsgp/clinical/gender-bias-in-medicine-and-medical-research-is-st.

4. Hogenboom, M. 2021, 'The hidden load: How "thinking of everything" holds mums back', retrieved from www.bbc.com/worklife/article/20210518-the-hidden-load-how-thinking-of-everything-holds-mums-back.

5. Anderson, A. (n.d.), 'A metaphor can open a doorway into your mind', retrieved from https://lifecoachadele.com/metaphor-doors-psyche/.

6. Van Agteren, J., Iasiello, M., Lo, L., Bartholomaeus, J., Kopsaftis, Z., Carey, M. and Kyrios, M. 2021, 'A systematic review and meta-analysis of psychological interventions to improve mental wellbeing', *Nature Human Behaviour*, 5(5), pp. 631–52.

7. Shutterfly Community 2019, '55+ Strong women quotes to inspire you', retrieved from www.shutterfly.com/ideas/strong-women-quotes/.

Chapter 1

1. 'What is mental health?' (n.d.), retrieved 17 August 2022 from www.beyondblue.org.au/the-facts/what-is-mental-health.

2. Ackerman, C. 2018, 'Life satisfaction theory and four contributing factors (+ scale)', retrieved 13 November 2022 from https://positivepsychology.com/life-satisfaction.

3. Iasiello, M., Van Agteren, J. and Cochrane, E. M. 2020.

4. 'Resilience' (n.d.), retrieved 17 August 2022 from www.apa.org/topics/resilience.

5. Lessard, K. 2022, 'What is "Flourishing"? Learn how to walk the 5-part path to happiness (at work)', retrieved 30 July 2022 from www.linkedin.com/pulse/what-flourishing-learn-how-walk-5-part-path-happiness-kylee-lessard/.

6. Kitchener, B.A., Jorm, A.F. and Kelly, C.M. 2017, *Mental Health First Aid Manual* (4th ed.), Mental Health First Aid Australia, Melbourne, p. 4.

7. Kitchener, B.A., Jorm, A.F. and Kelly, C.M. 2017.

8. Iasiello, M., Van Agteren, J., and Cochrane, E. M. 2020.

9. 'Depression', retrieved 17 August 2022 from https://www.who.int/news-room/fact-sheets/detail/depression.

10. Astbury, J. 2001, 'Gender disparities in mental health', Mental health. Ministerial Round Tables 54th World Health Assemble, WHO, Geneva, Switzerland.

11. 'Mental disorders', retrieved 17 August 2022 from www.who.int/news-room/fact-sheets/detail/mental-disorders.

12. Regis College, 'Women's mental health 101: Statistics, symptoms & resources,' retrieved 8 November 2022 from https://online.regiscollege.edu/blog/womens-mental-health/.

13. World Health Organization. (n.d.), 'Gender disparities in mental health', retrieved from www.who.int/mental_health/media/en/242.pdf.

14. Mooney-Somers, J., Deacon, R.M., Anderst, A. et al. 2020, 'Women in contact with the Sydney LGBTIQ communities: Report of the SWASH lesbian, bisexual and queer women's health survey 2016, 2018, 2020', Sydney Health Ethics, University of Sydney, p. 2.

15. 'Women and Mental Health', 2017, retrieved 17 August 2022 from https://psychology.org.au/inpsych/2017/february/fisher.

16. 'Women's Mental Health' (n.d.), https://homewoodhealth.com/corporate/blog/womens-mental-health.

17. Dawel, A., Shou, Y., Smithson, M. et al. 2020, 'The effect of COVID-19 on mental health and wellbeing in a representative sample of Australian adults', *Frontiers in Psychiatry*, 11, https://doi.org/10.3389/fpsyt.2020.579985.

18. 'Women's Health Survey', retrieved 13 November 2022 from www.jeanhailes.org.au/research/womens-health-survey/survey2022.

19. Davidson, M. 2012, *A Nurse's Guide to Women's Mental Health*, Springer Publishing, New York, p. 4.

20. Davidson, M. 2012, p. 3.

21. Durand, V., Barlow, D. and Hofmann, S. 2019, *Essentials of Abnormal Psychology*, (8th ed.), Cengage Learning, Inc., p. 33.

22. Srivastava, K. 2012, 'Women and mental health: Psychosocial perspective', *Industrial Psychiatry Journal*, 21(1), pp. 1–3.

23. Castle, D. and Abel, K. (eds). 2016, *Comprehensive: Women's mental health*, Cambridge University Press, Cambridge.

24. Rickwood, D.J. and Thomas K.A. 2019, 'Mental wellbeing interventions: An evidence check rapid review brokered by the Sax Institute for VicHealth', retrieved 13 November 2022 from www.saxinstitute.org.au/evidence-check/mental-wellbeing-interventions/.

25. Perry, B. and Winfrey, O. 2021, *What Happened to You? Conversations on trauma, resilience, and healing*, Flatiron Books, London, p. 75.

26. Hari, J. 2018, *Lost Connections: Uncovering the real causes of depression — and the unexpected solutions*, Bloomsbury Circus, London, p. 42.

27. 'Women and Mental Health', retrieved 13 November 2022 from www.nimh.nih.gov/health/topics/women-and-mental-health.

28. McKeever, N. 2021, 'Process Based Therapy: An introduction', retrieved from https://theweekenduniversity.com/process-based-therapy-introduction/.

29. McKeever, N.

30. Perry, B. and Winfrey, O. 2021, p. 17.

31. Perry, B. and Winfrey, O. 2021, p. 92.

32. Tran, D. 2018, 'National health survey of women reveals many feel anxious or are clinically depressed', retrieved from www.abc.net.au/news/2018-09-01/national-health-survey-australian-women-anxious-depressed/10188498#:~:text=66.9%20per%20cent%20of%20women,themselves%20on%20a%20weekly%20basis.

Chapter 2

1. Harris, R. 2009, *ACT Made Simple: An easy-to-read primer on acceptance and commitment therapy*, Harbinger Publications, Oakland, p. 8.

2. Siegel, D.J. 2007, *The Mindful Brain: Reflection and attunement in the cultivation of wellbeing*, WW Norton and Company, New York, p 31.

3. Lessard, K. 2022.

4. Frederickson, B. 2009, *Positivity: Groundbreaking research to release your inner optimist and thrive*, Oneworld, Oxford, p.32.

5. 'Decades of Scientific Research that Started a Growth Mindset Revolution' (n.d.). retrieved 17 August 2022 from www.mindsetworks.com/science/.

6. Mlodinow, L. 2022, *Emotional: The new thinking about feelings*, Penguin, p. 43.

7. Mlodinow, L. 2022, p. 35.

8. 'Paul Eckman', retrieved 17 August 2022 from www.goodtherapy.org/famous-psychologists/paul-ekman.html.

9. Gu, S., Wang, F., Patel, N.P., Bourgeois, J.A. and Huang, J.H. 2019, 'A model for basic emotions using observations of behaviour in drosophila', (review), *Frontiers in Psychology*, 10, https://doi.org/10.3389/fpsyg.2019.00781.

10. Brown, B. 2021, *Atlas of the Heart: Mapping meaningful connection and the language of human experience*, Vermilion, London, pp. ix–x.

11. Cherry, K. 'What is empathy?' retrieved 19 August 2022 from https://verywellmind.com/what-is-empathy-2795562.

12. Brown, B. 2021, p. 13.

13. Fogg, B.J. 2020, *Tiny Habits: Why starting small makes lasting change easy*, Penguin, London, p. 12.

14. McKay, S. 2018, *The Women's Brain Book: The neuroscience of health, hormones and happiness*, Hachette Australia, Sydney, p. 65.

15. Seppala, E. 2012, 'Connect to Thrive: Social connection improves health, wellbeing, longevity,' retrieved from www.psychologytoday.com/au/blog/feeling-it/201208/connect-thrive.

16. Hanson, R. 2013, *Hardwiring Happiness: The new brain science of contentment, calm and confidence*, Rider Books, London.

17. Mlodinow, L. 2022, p. 141.

18. Howes, L. 2022, 'Brain surgeon reveals how to heal trauma and destroy negative thoughts! Dr Rahul Jandial', retrieved from https://youtu.be/JYalx8bvEyg.

19. Al Taher, R. 2016, 'The classification of character strengths and virtues', retrieved from https://positivepsychology.com/classification-character-strengths-virtues/#women-strengths.

20. Neff, K. 2003, 'Self-compassion: An alternative conceptualisation of a healthy attitude toward oneself', *Self and Identity*, 2, p. 86.

21. Neff, K. 2021, *Fierce Self-Compassion: How women can harness kindness to speak up, claim their power and thrive*, Penguin Life, London, p. 6.

22. Neff, K.D., and Germer, C.K. 2013, 'A pilot study and randomized controlled trial of the mindful self-compassion program', *Journal of Clinical Psychology*, 69(1), pp. 28–44.

23. Steidl, S. 2020, *The Gift of Compassion: How to understand and overcome suffering*, Australian Academic Press, Samford Valley, p. 7.

24. Neff, K. 2021, p. 20.

25. Neff, K. 2021, p. 173.

26. Corey, G. 2020, Theory and Practice of Counselling and Psychotherapy, 10th ed., Cengage Learning, US, p. 130.

27. Dakin, B (interview), 'The hardest things we do in life might bring us the most meaning', Therapytips.org, 24 July 2022, reported in Travers, M. 'How to Bring Deeper Meaning into Your Life: Research clearly shows that it's tied to a desire to help others'.

28. Winn, M. 2014, 'What is your Ikigai?' retrieved 5 December 2017 from http://theviewinside.me/what-is-your-ikigai/.

29. Allen, S. 2019, 'How thinking about the future makes life more meaningful', retrieved 18 August 2022 from www.mindful.org/how-thinking-about-the-future-makes-life-more-meaningful/.

30. Frederickson, B. 2009, p.187.

31. Kitchener, B.A., Jorm, A.F. and Kelly, C.M. 2017, p. 48.

Chapter 3

1. 'My biggest opponent was inside my head: Exclusive book extract', *Sunday Mail*, retrieved 30 October 2022, p. 28.

2. Neff, K. 2003, pp. 85–101.

3. Brown, B. 2007, *I Thought it Was Just Me (But it Isn't)*, Avery, New York, p. 18.

4. Hari, J. 2018, p. 92.

5. Howell, C. 2016, *Listening, Learning, Caring & Counselling*, Exisle Publishing, Wollombi, p. 132.

6. Harris, R. 2010, *The Confidence Gap: From fear to freedom*, Exisle Publishing, Wollombi, p. 69.

7.   Harris, R. 2009, *ACT Made Simple: A quick-start guide to ACT basics and beyond*, New Harbinger Publications, Oakland, p. 2.

8.   Neff, K. 2003.

9.   Neff, K.D. and Germer, C.K. (in press), 'A pilot study and randomized controlled trial of the Mindful Self-Compassion Program,' *Journal of Clinical Psychology*.

10. Steidl, S. 2020, p. 7.

11. Steidl, S. 2020, p. 149.

12. Brown, B. 2007, p. 32.

13. Fredrickson, B. 2009, p. 209.

14. Steidl, S. 2020, p. 151.

15. Steidl, S. 2020, p. 157–9.

16. Harris, R. 2010, p 19.

Chapter 4

1.   Moore, C. 2021, 'Embrace your circle of influence', retrieved from www.epinsight.com/post/embracing-your-circle-of-influence.

2.   Yuile, T. 2019, 'Overcome fear and anxiety with the AWARE technique', retrieved 20 October 2022 from https://wellingtonlifecoaching.co.nz/freedom-from-anxiety-aware-technique/.

3.   Harris, R. 2009, pp. 12–13.

4.   Harris, R. 2009.

5.   Harris, R. 2009, p. 20.

6.   Harris, R. 2009, p. 20.

7.   Harris, R. 2009, p. 137.

8.   'How to use STOPP', retrieved 17 August 2022 from www.getselfhelp.co.uk/stopp.htm.

9.   Harris, R. 2019, 'How to Drop Anchor,, retrieved from https://survivorsofabuserecovering.ca/wp-content/uploads/2019/10/Dropping-anchor-handout-ACE-formula-Russ-Harris-2019.pdf.

Chapter 5

1.   Fielding, S. 2021, 'Languishing is the mood of 2021. How to identify it and how to cope', retrieved from www.verywellmind.com/languishing-is-the-mood-of-2021-518099.

2. Cambridge Dictionary, 'Change', retrieved from https://dictionary.cambridge.org/dictionary/english/.

3. Thibaut, F. and van Wijngaarden-Cremers, P. 2020, 'Women's mental health in the time of COVID-19 pandemic', (mini review) *Frontiers in Global Women's Health*, 1, https://doi.org/10.3389/fgwh.2020.588372.

4. Lindsay, T. 2022, *The Certainty Myth: How to be resilient when the world keeps changing*, Exisle Publishing, Wollombi, p. 115.

5. White, M. 1995, 'Naming abuse and breaking from its effects', *Re-authoring Lives: Interviews and essays*, Dulwich Centre Publications, Adelaide, pp. 82–111.

6. Parker, G., Tavella, G. and Eyers, K. 2021, *Burnout: A guide to identifying burnout and pathways to recovery*, Allen & Unwin, Crows Nest, p. 3.

7. Parker, G., Tavella, G. and Eyers, K. 2021, p. 43.

8. Parker, G., Tavella, G. and Eyers, K. 2021, 141.

9. Parker, G., Tavella, G. and Eyers, K. 2021, p. 49.

10. Parker, G., Tavella, G. and Eyers, K. 2021, 115.

11. Parker, G., Tavella, G. and Eyers, K. 2021, p. 88.

12. Parker, G., Tavella, G. and Eyers, K. 2021, p. 161.

13. Media release:,11 December 2018, 'Prepare your mind, not just your house, for disaster this summer', https://psychology.org.au/about-us/news-and-media/media-releases/2018/prepare-your-mind,-not-just-your-house,-for-disast.

14. RACGP, 2013, 'Managing emergencies and pandemics in general practice: A guide for preparation, response and recovery', p. 32.

15. Thibaut, F. and van Wijngaarden-Cremers, P. 2020.

Chapter 6

1. APA Dictionary of Psychology, 'Mood', retrieved from https://dictionary.apa.org/mood.

2. Kitchener, B.A., Jorm, A.F. and Kelly, C.M. 2017, p. 22.

3. Black Dog Institute, (n.d). 'Facts and figures about mental health', retrieved from www.blackdoginstitute.org.au/wp-content/uploads/2020/04/1-facts_figures.pdf.

4. Castle, D. and Abel, K. 2016.

5. American Psychiatric Association 2013, *Diagnostic and Statistical*

Manual of Mental Disorders (5th ed.), https://doi.org/10.1176/appi.
books.9780890425596.

6. American Psychiatric Association 2013.

7. Segal, Z., Williams, J. and Teasdale, J. 2002, *Mindfulness Based Cognitive Therapy for Depression :A new approach to preventing relapse*, Guilford Press, New York.

8. Howell, C. and Murphy, M. 2011, *Release Your Worries: A guide to letting go of stress and anxiety*, Exisle Publishing, Wollombi, p. 194.

9. Brown, B. 2012, *Daring Greatly: How the courage to be vulnerable transforms the way we live, love, parent, and lead*, Penguin Books, London.

10. Lerner, D. 2022, 'Attachment grief: Living with the loss of a child', *Psychotherapy Networker*, 46(4) pp. 25–9.

11. Howell, C. 2016, pp. 190–1.

12. Smith, J. 2022, *Why Has Nobody Told Me This Before?*, Penguin Random House, London, p. 146.

13. White, C. and Denborough D. 1988, *Introduction to Narrative Therapy: A collection of practice-based writings*, Dulwich Centre Publications, Adelaide, p. 29.

14. Ryan, C. 2010, 'How hope therapy can get us through tough times', retrieved from https://www.alternet.org/story/146459/how_%22hope_therapy%22_can_get_us_through_tough_times.

15. The Wellbeing Team 2017, 'How hope can help manage stress', retrieved from www.wellbeing.com.au/mind-spirit/mind/Holding-on-to-hope.html.

16. Ryan, C. 2010.

17. Pegg, M. 2020, 'S is for Rick Snyder: His work on hope', retrieved from www.thepositiveencourager.global/h-rick-snyders-work-hope/.

Chapter 7

1. Brown, B. 2021, p. 33.

2. Selva, J. 2022, 'How to set healthy boundaries: 10 examples + PDF worksheets', retrieved from https://positivepsychology.com/great-self-care-setting-healthy-boundaries/.

3. Pourjali, F. and Zarnaghash, M. 2010, 'Relationships between assertiveness and the power of saying no with mental health among undergraduate student', *Procedia — Social and Behavioral Sciences*, 9, pp. 137–41.

4. Brown, B. 2021, p. 220.

5. Ravitch, S. 2020, 'Space between stimulus and response: Creating critical research paradises', www.methodspace.com/blog/space-between-stimulus-and-response-creating-critical-research-paradises.

6. O'Connor, R. 2001, *Active Treatment of Depression*, Norton, New York, p. 112.

7. Lim, M. 2018, 'Is loneliness Australia's next public health epidemic?' *InPsych*, 40(4) pp. 7–11.

8. Lim, M. 2018.

9. Winch, G. 2013, '10 Surprising facts about rejection. Research finds that rejection affects intelligence, reason and more', retrieved from www. psychologytoday.com/au/blog/the-squeaky-wheel/201307/10-surprising-facts-about-rejection.

10. Weir, K. 2012, 'The pain of social rejection: As far as the brain is concerned, a broken heart may not be so different to a broken arm,' *American Psychological Association*, 43(4), retrieved from www.apa.org/ monitor/2012/04/rejection.

11. McKay, M. and Wood, J. 2011, *The Dialectical Behaviour Therapy Diary: Monitoring your emotional regulation day by day*, New Harbinger Publications, Oakland.

12. Pederson, P. 2020, 'DBT skills-building card deck for clients and therapists', PESI Publishing and Media.

13. Pederson, P. 2020.

14. Vivyan, C. 2009, 'Unhelpful thinking habits', retrieved from www. getselfhelp.co.uk/docs/UnhelpulthinkingHabits with Alternavites.pdf.

15. McKay, M. and Wood, J. 2011.

16. McKay, M., Wood, J. and Brantley, J. 2019, *The Dialectical Behaviour Therapy Workbook: Practical DBT exercises for learning mindfulness, interpersonal effectiveness, emotion regulation and distress tolerance*, New Harbinger Publications, Oakland.

17. Ellen, S. and Deveny, C. 2018, *Mental: Everything you never knew you needed to know about mental health*, Black Inc., Carlton, p. 157.

18. Life in Mind, 2019, 'Suicide facts and stats', retrieved from www. lifeinmindaustralia.com.au/about-suicide/suicide-data/suicide-facts-and-stats.

19. Zetterqvist, M. 2015, 'The DSM-5 diagnosis of nonsuicidal self-injury disorder: A review of the empirical literature', *Child and Adolescent Psychiatry and Mental Health*, 9(1), 31.

20. Mental Health First Aid Australia 2017, 'Mental health first aid guidelines', retrieved from https://mhfa.com.au/mental-health-first- aid-guidelines.

21. Westers, N., Muehlenkamp, N. and Lau, M. 2016, 'SOARS model of risk assessment in non-suicidal self-injury', *Contemporary Paediatrics*, 33(7), pp. 25–31.

22. Mental Health First Aid Australia 2017.

23. Commonwealth of Australia, 2007, 'Foundations for effective practice: Square suicide questions answers resources', www.square.org.au/wp-content/uploads/sites/10/2013/05/Foundations-of-Effective-Practice_May2013.pdf

24. Ellen, S. and Deveny, C. 2018, p. 158.

25. Mental Health First Aid Australia 2017.

Chapter 8

1. 'About the menstrual cycle', retrieved 24 October 2022 from www.jeanhailes.org.au/health-a-z/periods/about-the-menstrual-cycle#what-is-a-menstrual-cycle.

2. Watson, S. 'Stages of the menstrual cycle,' retrieved 24 October 2022 from www.healthline.com/health/womens-health/stages-of-menstrual-cycle#luteal.

3. Skovlund, C.W., Mørch, L.S., Kessing, L.V. and Lidegaard, Ø. 2016, 'Association of hormonal contraception with depression', *JAMA Psychiatry*, 73(11), pp. 1154–62.

4. Kulkarni, J. 2020, 'Premenstrual dysphoric disorder', *Australian Doctor*, September.

5. Bloch, S., Green, S., Janca, A., Mitchell, P.B. and Robertson., M. 2017, *Foundations of Clinical Psychiatry*, Melbourne University Publishing, Melbourne, p. 420.

6. Kulkarni, J. 2020.

7. Kulkarni, J. 2020.

8. Panda (n.d.). 'Mental health and wellbeing during pregnancy,' retrieved 24 October 2022 from https://panda.org.au/articles/mental-health-and-wellbeing-during-pregnancy/.

9. Panda.

10. Bloch, M., Rotenberg, N., Koren, D. and Klein, E. 2005, 'Risk factors associated with the development of postpartum mood disorders', *Journal of Affective Disorders*, 88(1), pp. 9–18.

11. Fretts, R. C. and Spong, C. 2022, 'Stillbirth: Incidence, risk factors, etiology and prevention', retrieved 30 October 2022 from www.uptodate.com/contents/stillbirth-incidence-risk-factors-etiology-and-prevention.

12. Bloch, S., Green, S., Janca, A., Mitchell, P.B. and Robertson., M. 2017.

13. Danielson, K. 2020, 'Important facts about miscarriage,' retrieved 30 October 2022 from www.verywellfamily.com/miscarriage-facts-2371810.

14. University of Rochester Medical Center 2011, 'Women who miscarry have long-lasting mental health problems', retrieved 24 October 2022 from www.urmc.rochester.edu/news/story/women-who-miscarry-have-long-lasting-mental-health-problems.

15. Campbell-Jackson, L. and Horsch, A. 2014, 'The psychological impact of stillbirth on women: A systematic review', *Illness, Crisis & Loss*, 22(3), pp. 237–56.

16. Ezzel, W. 2016, 'The impact of infertility on women's mental health', *North Carolina Medical Journal*, 77(6): pp. 427–8.

17. Klemetti, R., Raitanen, J., Sihvo, S., Saarni, S. and Koponen, P. 2010, 'Infertility, mental disorders and wellbeing — a nationwide survey', *Acta Obstetricia et Gynecologica Scandinavica*, 89, pp. 677–82.

18. Mallorqui, A, et al. (2022), 'Anhedonia in endometriosis: An unexplored symptom', *Front Psychol*, 13, 935349. DOI: 10.3389/fpsyg.2022.945349.

19. Hoggenmueller, C. 'Menopause,' retrieved 22 October 2022 from https://drcarolineh.com/patients/menopause/.

20. Safro, E., Baber, R., & Magraith, K. (2022). 'Perimenopause.' Online course, Australasian Menopause Society.

21. Mitchell, J., 30 March 2021, 'What's your wellbeing plan?' retrieved 23 January 2023 from https://themindroom.com.au/whats-your-wellbeing-plan/.

22. Malone, S. and Weiss-Wolf, J. 2022, 'America lost its way on menopause research. It's time to get back on track', retrieved 22 October 2022 from www.washingtonpost.com/opinions/2022/04/28/menopause-hormone-therapy-nih-went-wrong/.

23. Australasian Menopause Society 2022, 'The 2022 hormone therapy position statement of the North American menopause society', retrieved 30 October 2022 from www.menopause.org.au/hp/position-statements/the-2022-hormone-therapy-position-statement-of-the-north-american-menopause-society.

24. Steiner, M., Dunn, E. and Born, L. 2003, 'Hormones and mood: From

menarche to menopause and beyond', Journal of Affective Disorders, 74(1), pp. 67–83.

Chapter 9

1. Chapman, G. 1992, *The 5 Love Languages: The secret to love that lasts*, Northfield Publishing, Chicago, p. 37.

2. Gottman, J. and Silver, N. 2007, *The Seven Principles for Making Marriage Work*, Orion Books, London, p. 79.

3. Harris, R. 2009, *ACT with Love: Stop struggling, reconcile differences, and strengthen your relationship with Acceptance and Commitment Therapy*, New Harbinger Publications, Oakland, p. 181.

4. Harris, R. 2009, p. 36.

5. Howell, C. 2020, *The Changing Man: A mental health guide*, Exisle Publishing, Wollombi, p. 181.

6. Harris, R. 2009, p. 131.

7. Harris, R. 2009.

8. Gottman, J. and Silver, N. 2007, p. 260.

9. Howell, C. 2020, pp. 196–7.

10. Whitbourne, S. 2017, 'The secret reason why sex is so crucial in relationships', retrieved August 2019 from www.psychologytoday.com/au/blog/fulfillment-any-age/201707.the-secret-reason-why-sex-is-so-crucial-in-relationships.

11. Stritof, S. 2020, '5 Common types of affairs', retrieved March 2020 from www.verywellmind.com/marriage-affair-2303083.

12. Castle, D. and Abel, K. 2016, p. 161.

13. United Nations 1993, 'General assembly declaration on the elimination of violence against women', retrieved 5 November 2022 from www.un-documents.net/a48r104.htm.

14. RACGP 2021, 'Abuse and violence — Working with our patients in general practice' (5th ed.), p. 23.

15. Castle, D. and Abel, K. 2016, p. 163.

16. Castle, D. and Abel, K. 2016, p. 2.

17. Relationships Australia 2017, 'Women and separation: Managing new horizons', retrieved 5 November 2022 from www.rasa.org.au/wp-content/uploads/2013/05/Women-Separation-W16029.pdf, p. 25.

18. RACGP 2021, p. 25.

19. RACGP 2021, p. 42.

20. American Psychiatric Association 2013, p. 646.

21. Casabianca, S.S. 2021, 'All about narcissistic personality disorder', retrieved 7 November 2022 from https://psychcentral.com/disorders/narcissistic-personality-disorder.

22. Better Help Editorial Team 2022, 'In a relationship with a narcissist? The 6 narcissistic love patterns to look for', retrieved 5 November 2022 from www.betterhelp.com/advice/love/are-you-in-a-relationship-with-a-narcissist-here-are-6-narcissistic-love-patterns-to-watch-out-for/.

23. Sander, S., Strizzi, J.M., Øverup, C.S., Cipric, A. and Hald, G.M. 2020, 'When love hurts: Mental and physical health among recently divorced Danes', *Frontiers in Psychology*, 11, https://doi.org/10.3389/fpsyg.2020.578083.

24. MentalHelp.net (n.d.), 'Emotional coping and divorce', retrieved 5 November 2022 from www.mentalhelp.net/divorce/emotional-coping/.

25. Relationships Australia 2017.

26. Holton, S., Fisher, J. and Rowe, H. 2010, 'Motherhood: Is it good for women's mental health?' *Journal of Reproductive and Infant Psychology*, 28(3), pp. 223–39.

27. Molgora, S. and Accordini, M. 2020, 'Motherhood in the time of coronavirus: The impact of the pandemic emergency on expectant and postpartum women's psychological wellbeing', *Frontiers in Psychology*, 11, 567155, https://doi.org/10.3389/fpsyg.2020.567155.

Chapter 10

1. RANZCP, 2020, 'Trauma informed practice', retrieved 8 November 2022, www.ranzcp.org/news-policy/policy-and-advocacy/position-statements/trauma-informed-practice.

2. World Health Organization 2013 'Global and regional estimates of violence against women. Prevalence and health effects of intimate partner violence and non-partner sexual violence', retrieved from www.who.int/publications/i/item/9789241564625.

3. Centre for Disease Control and Prevention 2022, 'Fast facts: Preventing sexual violence', retrieved 10 November 2022 from www.cdc.gov/violenceprevention/sexualviolence/fastfact.html.

4. Olff, M. 2017, 'Sex and gender differences in post-traumatic stress disorder: An update', *European Journal of Psychotraumatology*, 8, 1351204. https://doi.org/10.1080/20008198.2017.1351204.

5. Su, W. and Stone, L. 2020, 'Adult survivors of childhood trauma: Complex trauma, complex needs', *Australian Journal of General Practice*, 49(7), pp. 423–30.

6. Castle, D. and Abel, K. 2016, p. 162.

7. Castle, D. and Abel, K. 2016, p. 3.

8. Hughes, K., Bellis, M. A., Hardcastle, K. A., et al. 2017, 'The effect of multiple adverse childhood experiences on health: A systematic review and meta-analysis', *Lancet Public Health*, 2(8), pp. e356–66.

9. Su, W. and Stone, L. 2020.

10. Sweeton, J. 2019, 'Trauma treatment', PESI course, Wisconsin.

11. Van der Kolk, B. 2014, *The Body Keeps the Score: Brain, mind, and body in the healing of trauma*, Penguin Books, New York, p. 66.

12. Child Welfare Information Gateway 2015, 'Understanding the effects of maltreatment on brain development', retrieved July 2019 from www.childwelfare.gov/pubs/issue-briefs/brain-development.

13. Freedman, E. 2020, 'Clinical management of patients presenting following a sexual assault', *Australian Journal of General Practice*, 49(7), pp. 406–11.

14. Su, W. and Stone, L. 2020.

15. Tanasugarn, A. 2020, 'Is it Borderline Personality Disorder or is it really complex PTSD?' retrieved 15 August 2022 from www.psychologytoday.com/au/blog/understanding-ptsd/202006/is-it-borderline-personality-disorder-or-is-it-really-complex-ptsd.

16. World Health Organization 2019, 'International statistical classification of diseases and related health problems' (11th revision), https://icd.who.int/.

17. Hanson, R. 2013, *Hardwiring Happiness: The new brain science of contentment, calm and confidence*, Rider Books, London.

18. Van der Kolk, B. 2014, p. 68.

19. Sweeton, J. 2019.

20. Van der Kolk, B. 2014.

21. Sweeton, J. 2019.

22. Su, W. and Stone, L. 2020.

23. Scott, M. 2013, *CBT for Common Trauma Responses*, SAGE Publications Ltd, p. 63.
24. Harris, R. 2021, *Trauma-focused ACT: A practitioner's guide to working with mind, body and emotion using Acceptance and Commitment therapy*, New Harbinger, Oakland, p. 5.
25. Wingard, B., Johnson, C. and Drahm-Butler, T. 2015, *Aboriginal Narrative Practice: Honouring storylines of pride, strength and creativity*, Dulwich Centre Publications, Adelaide, p. 13.

Chapter 11

1. Australian Institute of Health and Welfare 2016, 'Illicit use of drugs', retrieved from www.aihw.gov.au/reports-data/behaviours-risk- factors/illicit-use-of-drugs/reports.
2. Ellen, S. & Deveny, C. 2018, p. 126.
3. Sinnerton, J. 2022, 'Stressed women binge drinking', *The Advertiser*.
4. Castle, D. and Abel, K. 2016, p. 178.
5. Howell, C. 2020, p. 115.
6. Ellen, S. and Deveny, C. 2018, p. 155.
7. Cunningham, M. 2019, 'Trapped in the Net: Are we all addicted to our smartphones?' retrieved from www.theage.com. au/national/victoria/trapped-in-the-net-are-we-all-addicted-to-our- smartphones-20190531-p51t44.html.
8. Smith, M., Robinson, L. and Segal, J. 2019, 'Smartphone addiction', retrieved July 2019 from www.helpguide.org/articles/ addictions/smartphone-addiction.htm.
9. Fox, D. 2021, *Complex Borderline Personality Disorder*, New Harbinger Publications, Oakland, p. 21.
10. Tanasugarn, A. 2020.
11. Casanova, E. and Casanova, M. 2019, *Defining Autism: A guide to brain, biology and behavior*, Jessica Kingsley Publishers, London, p. 43.
12. Bradshaw, P. and Pickett, C. 2021, 'Recognising, supporting and understanding Autistic adults in general practice settings', *Australian Journal of General Practice*, 50(3), pp. 126–30.
13. Crosby, B. and Lippert, T. 2006, *Transforming ADHD: Simple, effective attention and action regulation skills to help you focus and succeed*, New Harbinger Publications, Oakland, pp. 122–5.

14. Rowe, E. 2018, 'Early detection of eating disorders in general practice', *Australian Family Physician*, 46(11), pp. 833–8.
15. American Psychiatric Association 2013, p. 329.
16. Luck, A.J., Morgan, J.F., Reid, F., et al. 2002, 'The SCOFF questionnaire and clinical interview for eating disorders in general practice: Comparative study', *British Medical Journal*, 325(7367), pp. 755–6.
17. Kitchener, B.A., Jorm, A.F. and Kelly, C.M. 2017, p. 109.
18. Castle, D. and Abel, K. 2016, p. 197.
19. Butterfly. (n.d.) 'Can body image issues be serious?' retrieved 12 November 2022 from https://butterfly.org.au/body-image/can-body-image-issues-be-serious/.
20. American Psychiatric Association 2013, p. 242.
21. Butterfly (n.d.) 'Boosting body image', retrieved 12 November 2022 from https://butterfly.org.au/body-image/boosting-body-image/.
22. Kitchener, B.A., Jorm, A.F. and Kelly, C.M. 2017, p. 60.

Chapter 12

1. Bloch, S. and Green, S. (eds) 2017, *Foundations of Clinical Psychiatry* (4th ed.), Melbourne University Press, Melbourne, p. 432.
2. Acacia Connection, (n.d.), 'Positive ageing', retrieved 12 November 2022 from www.eapcounselling.com.au/wp-content/uploads/2018/10/Positive-Ageing.pdf.
3. Acacia Connection.
4. Boehm, J.K., Winning, A., Segerstrom, S. and Kubzansky, L.D. 2015, 'Variability modifies life satisfaction's association with mortality risk in older adults', *Psychological Science*, 26(7), pp. 1063–70.
5. Ai, A.L., Wink, P. and Ardelt, M. 2010, 'Spirituality and aging: A journey for meaning through deep interconnection in humanity', in J.C. Cavanaugh and C.K. Cavanaugh (eds), *Aging in America*, vol. 3. Societal issues, pp. 222–46.
6. Bloch, S. and Green, S. (eds) 2017, p. 444.
7. Bloch, S. and Green, S. (eds) 2017, p. 454.
8. Government of South Australia. (n.d.), 'What is elder abuse?' retrieved 12 November 2022 from www.sahealth.sa.gov.au/wps/wcm/connect/public+content/sa+health+internet/conditions/stop+elder+abuse/what+is+elder+abuse.

9. Szoeke, C. 2021, Secrets of Women's Healthy Ageing, Melbourne University Press, Melbourne, p. 13.

10. Stanton, A., Revenson, T. and Tennen, H. 2007, 'Health psychology: Psychological adjustment to chronic disease, *Annual Review of Psychology*, 58, 13, pp. 1–13.

11. Szoeke, C. 2021, p. 43.

12. White, K., Issac, M.S., Kamoun, C., Leygues J. and Cohn, S. 2018, 'The THRIVE model: A framework and review of internal and external predictors of coping with chronic illness', *Health Psychology Open*, 5(2), https://doi:10.1177/2055102918793552.

13. Hutchison, S., Clutton, S., Youl, P. and Chambers, S. 2011, 'Reducing the psychological impact of cancer for regional Queenslanders', *InPsych*, 33(5), retrieved 13 November 22 from https://psychology.org.au/for-members/publications/inpsych/2011/oct/reducing-the-psychosocial-impact-of-cancer-for-reg.

14. Sharma, S. 2020, 'International association for the study of pain (IASP) updates the definition of pain', JOSPT, retrieved from www.jospt.org/do/10.2519/jospt.blog.20200812/full/.

15. Wilson, H., Harris-Roxas, B., Lintzeris, N. and Harris, M. 2022, 'Diagnosing and managing patients with chronic pain who develop prescription opioid use disorder: A scoping review of general practitioners' experience', *Australian Journal of General Practice*, 51(10), pp. 804–11.

16. Bejot, Y., Brayne, C., Filip, I. et al. 2019, 'Estimation of the global prevalence of dementia in 2019 and forecasted prevalence in 2050: An analysis for the Global Burden of Disease Study 2019', Elsevier Ltd., retrieved 12 November 2022 from www.thelancet.com/journals/lanpub/article/PIIS2468-2667%2821%2900249-8/fulltext.

Final words on flourishing

1. Szoeke, C. 2021, p. 114.

2. www.personalgrowthcourses.net/stories/williamson.ourdeepestfear.invitation.

Index

126, 259–60
and loneliness 185
cravings, coping strategies 293–4
creativity, within relationships 238–9
criticism, effect of 67
Crosby, Greg 303

D

Dakin, Brodie 51
'date nights' 239
defusion process 105, 107–8
dementia
    common types 325
    early signs 325–6
    influences on 321
    treatment 326
Denise's story
    grief counselling 167–8
    onset of depression 139–40
    role of guilt 161
depression
    in the ageing 319–20, 321
    chemical messengers 137–8
    explained 135
    general experiences with 140–1
    management plan 145
    with menopause 224
    overcoming 157–8
    during perimenopause 222–3, 224
    questions about 153
    relapse prevention plan 159–60
    risk factors 138
    statistics 14
    symptoms 141
    understanding levels of 137–43
Dialectical Behaviour Therapy 188–90,
    192–4
Dickens, Charles 60
'dirty fighting' 237
disabilities, caused by abuse/violence
    248–9
disasters see natural disasters
disorganized attachment style 242
'distress tolerance box' 191
divorce
    multiple losses from 254–5
    strategies for managing 256–7

working through the grief 255
'Drop Anchor' technique 112
Dweck, Carol 30
dysthymia 142

E

eating disorders
    explained 304–5
    raising the issue 308
    signs and symptoms 305–6
    statistics 14, 304
    treatment 307–8
Eckman, Paul 36
Einstein, Albert 315
elder abuse 320
'emotion mind' 189
'emotional affairs' 246
emotional distress
    coping with 188–94
    relaxation skills 191
emotions
    be mindful of 34–8
    echoed by mood 135–7
    positive 73–4
    positive vs negative 35
empathy 37, 77–8
endometriosis 221
Estes, Clarise Pinkola 172
eustress 83
exercise 145–6
exposure, gradual 100
exposure technique 278
Eye Desensitization and Reprocessing
    279–80

F

facial expressions 36
'fair fighting' rules 237
'fawn' and 'flock' behaviour 89
feelings
    be mindful of 34–8
    managing 169–70
femicide 248
fight, flight or freeze response 88–9, 267
finding time 24
Fitzgerald, Ella 27
'five love languages' 231